Abundant Heart

Abundant Heart

THOUGHTS ON HEALING, LOVING, AND LIVING FREE

LAURA STALEY

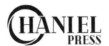

Abundant Heart: Thoughts on Healing, Loving, and Living Free
Laura Staley

Tradepaper ISBN: 978-1-945026-82-9
Electronic ISBN: 978-1-945026-83-6
Library of Congress Control Number: 2021943385

Published by Haniel Press
An Imprint of Sacred Stories Publishing, Fort Lauderdale, FL
Printed in the United States of America

For Ruby

Beautiful,
Loving Soul Twin

Table of Contents

SECTION TWO: QUIRKY

SECTION THREE: LOVE AND LOSS

SECTION FOUR: ABUNDANT HEART

SECTION FIVE: EXPANSIVE

RECLAIM

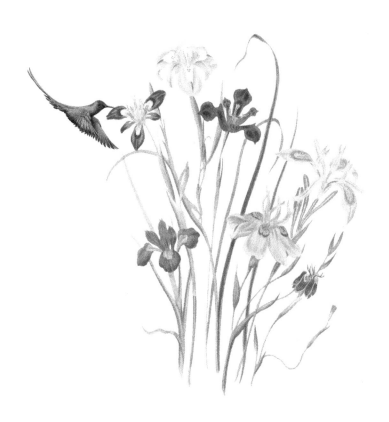

Impulsive

Some angels gathered before my soul came down to earth as I sat in the front row so eager to **go**. The angels said, "We've got a super, challenging assignment. Think long and hard about whether you want this particular life journey on planet earth."

I jumped out of my seat, hand waving up in the air.

"*Pick Me! Pick Me! Pick Me! Ooo! Ooo! Ooo!*"

I danced around like I needed a bio break.

The angels looked at me and said, "Really?!?! YOU?!?!?"

It had already begun. I realized I needed to be sitting in my seat, so I sat back down, yet squirmed with ecstatic excitement, my hand still waving in the air.

"*YES! ME! ME! ME! I CAN DO THIS!! I WANNA LIVE ON EARTH no matter how challenging, terrifying, or what happens to my earthly body, brain, heart, and psyche--I WANNA LIVE ON EARTH!*"

So, they sent my soul down to planet earth...

On earth, I've learned to sit quietly and ponder some things before I impulsively say "YES!"

And "OH MY GOSH," what serious training this continues to be! Those angels had been accurate, truthful-when they described how hard it would be...Wow! They forgot to let my soul know how incredibly beautiful it could be, too, with all kinds of things in-between places, the shoved together simultaneously things, like how a plate of food can have the eggs touching the toast; the crumbs of the toast get on the eggs, and the honey for the toast gets sticky all over everything on the plate, table, and my fingers.

A beloved one asked me yesterday, "Seriously, how have you come through all of that mayhem?"

I thought for a while. Rather than blurting out some words like "Courage" or "Feistiness" or "Willpower" or a whole string of Salty Sailor words, I listened to my heart which said, "I came through by returning to my center, the dynamic sweet spot of my Inner Fly on the Wall, the Experiencer of Life experiences, that grew into Inner Quiet Charlotte, a gazillion times in gratitude. I have anchored deep inside me an unwavering fierce optimism-a belief that Love Always Finds a Way to Love. I know that my soul came here to love and be loved in return. My soul is Love. I returned to Love every single time some shoe flew at my face, or my dog peed on the carpet, or the stars twinkled in the night sky.

Do you know why you came to planet earth? I hope you'll figure that out inside your own heart or wherever you go to figure things out.

I do know—

You are loved more than you can even imagine. You matter. Pain births wisdom. Cherish You.

Fulfilled

To laugh at yourself and life's foibles,
To endure all types of traumas
And to rise strong with a quiet mind, a loving heart,
And a peaceful countenance.
To welcome the honesty of beloved ones,
To walk away from those who would break your spirit,
To forgive the seemingly unforgivable,
To accept the seemingly unacceptable,
To cultivate compassion,
To know you matter,
To delight in the beautiful,
To seek the best in others,
To uplift the world with your gifts, courage, truths, and
lessons learned.
To experience fearlessness even for a day
To leave the world with soft love handprints
on people's hearts,
A glorious flower or vegetable garden,
A home as a safe haven of love,
A vibrant, thriving child,
A dance, a recipe, or crafty creation.

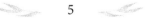

To know in your soul that you left it all on the field with everything you had,

To know even one person grew, breathed,
laughed, and felt valued,
Because you lived.
This embodies a fulfilled life.

Cherish You

I have learned that other people's judgments and criticisms rarely have anything to do with me. Their condemnations come from unresolved hurts, the person's inner critic, shame-maker, or straight-jacketed unexamined expectation machine. I've learned that some individuals will not ever approve of or accept me or my choices, ever. I'm at peace with that. I've learned that other people are moved by the Dignity, Love, and Compassion I have become because that Dignity, Love, and Compassion lives inside them.

When I live aligned with my deepest values and take actions from my Inner Wisdom, I no longer require applause or fear the disdain or the dismissal of other people. All these reactions from others probably will happen. All these reactions of other people remain out of my control, forever and always.

I continue to make myself right with mySelf from the inside, the anchors of post-traumatic wisdom, confidence, grace, compassion, dignity, joy, and honor. I no longer fear the inner self-loathing because she's become silent and was not my Voice, anyway. When I make mistakes, I own them and learn from them. I forgive myself and change some more behaviors.

I am free to set boundaries. I can say, "No, thank you." I can live true to my core values. I live free to be a humane human being.

Valuable

*W*hen difficult things happened in my life, I used to think that it was my fault. I was not a good enough person. I wasn't grateful enough for all the blessings in my life, including the hard things. I wasn't a smart enough student of life to figure out the secret practices to keep me safe from heartbreak. I thought I still carried around too many limiting beliefs in my unconscious including some of the following: life loved kicking me; I got punished for being crabby to the people I loved the most; I got triggered as a way for me to discern a thousand ways I could either react or respond that often finally included laughing; the stupid mistakes I made twenty years ago or yesterday flew back to smack me in the face.

Conversely, when beautiful, loving miracles of kindness and tenderness spontaneously happened, out of the black and blue, I thought I had absolutely nothing to do with those gifts. I hadn't earned them. I wasn't worthy of their appearance in my life. I could barely breathe them into my heart.

I've learned to share love and kindness generously from my heart and to receive love no matter what happens in the realm of external realities. I discovered that anchors sink into the inside, not the outside. Protection from life events does not exist. The way I respond to circumstances shifts the trajectory of my life from the inside out.

Is the butterfly loved because its wings flutter? Does the gosling wonder if it's eating the grass the correct way, too much or too little? Does the wind worry where its next paycheck comes from? Are you as valuable as a tree, a ruler, a bowl of blueberries, a red cardinal? Where does worthiness live? What contains the measure of your or another person's life? What does it mean to be valuable? Are you loved for existing?

Here Now

I sit seemingly between two worlds.
One I knew, endured
And this one
Created each day I
Wake up vibrantly
Still present.

I notice a pattern of
Intermittent
Weepy tears of gratitude.

This soul of mine
Cleanses the past,
Misses people I love,
Feels free, safe to
Express joy in being alive
When many have died,
Are dying, struggling, suffering in
Countless ways.

Who am I to be full of life?
Who am I not to be?

Always in my heart,
You are.
Love.
Create.
Me.
We.
Here.
Now.

Fearshame

Got distance from
You
That held me
Frozen in my tracks.
I hear you
A hidden, terrifying, poisonous
Constrictor
Lurking, silently
Awaiting
the
Death of possibilities.

Suffocating
Potential
Airways,
Passageways for
Freedom.

You attempted to
Convince me I could

Not move, grow, heal,
Transform.

You tricked me
Into believing
That you were me,
That I was you.

I suddenly see you,
A snake
Separate from Love's Truth.

From a deep river
Of hot belly water
You
Slither
Far, far away
For now.

A Big Question

How do you want your body touched?
Did you even know
You could tell people
Your preferences or did you
Feel like an object passed around?
Swatted,
Spanked,
Smacked,
Grabbed,
Pinched,
Bruised,
Punched,
Shoved
Defiled by larger humans
Entitled to
Your girl parts.

Touch

Did not know
This body
Was not an
Object for others
To poke, squeeze,
Smack, spank,
Startle, shock,
Molest.
Did not know
This voice
Could tell him
"NO!" and
He would still
Persist in proceeding.
"No!" did not
Ever mean "Yes."
"No" always meant
Stop what you
Are doing with
Your hands, arms,
Chest, mouth,

Cockadoodle Do.
Freeze frame
This Instance!
Hear these
Preferences for
Gentle, soft, tender
Touch,
For a Love
Connection.
Affection does not equal
A sexual pursuit agenda goal
Of Getting Off all over.
A French kiss is not
A predetermined gateway to
A Baseball Game of
Tagging the bases of
This body!
My lady parts are not bags
Placed on a dusty, muddy
Field of Dreams
Made for Your
Landslide into
Home Plate.
When did sexual
Interactions become a
Strong-armed
Transaction rather than a
Spiritual Revelation?
Whole people await

Acceptance,
Love.
Creation.
My
Skin,
Humanity
Remain
Steadfast
Exuding
Internal
Reverence.

Reframe That Game

You taught
Us tricks,
Songs,
And silly rhymes.
I felt safe
At parades
Family picnics
And
Swimming pools.

I watched you
With mug and brush,
Strap and blade
Shave your silver
Whiskers.
All those old
School tools.

Leaning up to
Kiss your cheek.
Smelling of

Old Spice
You seemed
Nonplussed
And I
Quite meek.

Then it happened
That one time
Exchange
I kept it shrouded,
Silent.
An internal pain.

I've done my work
And healed
This past.
I ask myself
Now, could I
Reframe?

I'm nine years old
You stand
There asking
Me,
"Play and pet
My
One eyed
Trouser Mouse."

Surprised, I ask,
Don't you
Want to do
This activity
With another louse?

I don't think
This is Parcheesi,
Spades, or Go Fish.
Your pockets
Remain empty of
Horehound deelish.

When I ask about
Your wife,
You tell me,
"You are beautiful
And she is not."
Seriously?
I look like a boy
Without the parts.

Put
Your mouse
Back in its house!
Find someone
Your own age
To play this
Odd game of

Hearts.
You are
Dead now.
You died years
Ago.

Your secret shame
Remained With
Me until
This final
Lyrical
Heave Ho.

I love
And forgive you
For you did not
Know what to do
With your status
Your pain and
Twisted desire.

Embracing my
Beauty took
Years of unfolding
I'm here now
Radiant,
Glowing,
A Super Nova
Full of fire.

Sacred Haven

Right here
In Large
Strong
Warm
Arms
I will
Cuddle
Hold
Soothe
You.

Light
Fingers
Gently
Caress
Your
Face
Touching your
Wet, salty
Tears of fear with
Quiet knowing.

Curl up
In this wide
Soft luxurious
Lap of
Kindness
A comforting,
Cozy
Fluffy blanket of
Acceptance
Grace.

For I
Am with
You always
The safe
Haven
Your
Tender
Silent
Soul
Within.

Isolation Leads to Loving Connection

At 14 years old, after a mental meltdown, the first of many types of spiritual awakenings I would experience, I lived for one month in solitary confinement. I surrendered all my clothing and eyeglasses in exchange for a thick, scratchy-like burlap, short-sleeved green covering. This garment felt nothing like a gown.

I experienced a constant bone-cold chill inside that all-white room. A thin mattress and one blanket did not prove to provide much warmth. Because I had extreme myopia, the staff appeared blurry; ghostlike blobs, entering the room to bring trays of food. In my efforts to orient myself to this altered reality, I engaged all my senses even beyond the five we are constantly told we have. These additional senses include: interoception-the ability to sense ones' internal body-the tightening of muscles, the expansion of the lungs, visceroception-the ability to sense body signals such as hunger and thirst, and proprioception-the ability to sense one's body in relationship to the surroundings such as the floor beneath one's feet.

I will never forget the sound of keys jangling, signaling a human being was approaching who would soon be unlocking doors, including the one that opened to where I sat, moved, ate, and slept. I faced three doors-one to freedom, one to restraints, and one to the bathroom. Like the game show on TV with Monty Hall, I always wanted to choose the door to my freedom. I began to discover that one's freedom remains on the inside, the work with one's thoughts, feelings, intuition, imagination, and internal sensations.

I vividly remember the scent of grape bubble gum of the staff member whose energy felt consistently kind. When she managed to get close enough, I noticed her long, thick, straight black Cher-like hair. Another staff member repeatedly yelled at me. Filled with anger, she interrogated me with, "Do you know why you are here?"

Because I never knew the answer to that question, I did not speak. I figured out that my parents placed me in the psyche hospital and pieced together why they took that action. Yet, I never knew why I got put in solitary confinement. The question, "Do you know why you're here?" became an existential question that I continue to ponder. Even this morning, I asked myself, "Laura, do you know why you are here?" Fortunately, I eventually collaged an answer together that continues to turn a bit--kind of like looking through a dazzling, colorful kaleidoscope.

Once released from solitary confinement, I interacted with my other bin mates (a term I created). I befriended a young man who loved playing his harmonica.

The staff let us know that a talent show would be happening soon. Staff encouraged us to sign up because both staff and bin mates were welcome to participate. I urged my friend to sign-up. I let him know that he played the harmonica with great skill and passion. I loved listening to him play and told him so. He kept saying he wasn't good enough to play in the talent show. He did not believe in his talent, his gifts. I continued to encourage him. I knew in my heart that he played well, that his musical talent deserved recognition.

One day I looked at the sign-up sheet and spotted his name. I felt much joy. When I saw him later that day, I gave him a big hug. He began calling me his Lil' Con Artist.

The day arrived for the talent show, and I sat right next to my friend. His hands shook. I kept smiling over at him, looking into his eyes with reassurance, and whispered, "I believe in you." His turn to perform came. He walked to the front of the room. He played his harmonica with all his heart and soul. When he completed, the room erupted. Everyone rose to their feet, cheering loudly, clapping, chanting his name. Tears streamed down his face as he received our love, our appreciation. We cheered louder.

The gifts that I gleaned from these experiences include a keen ability to notice people's energy states even if their mouths fake smile at me or their spoken words tell lies about their true gifts and passions. I notice people light up when talking about their joys. I observe when people are completely busy in their heads and not grounded in their bodies. I know all these experiences in myself.

Every cell of my body knows that nothing replaces the in-person acceptance, kindness, rapt attention-listening, loving hugs, tenderness, discernment, grace, honesty, curiosity, compassionate energy presence of another human being. Nothing.

You have more than five senses and some of you have cultivated a keen inner emotional guidance system alongside proprioception, visceroception, and interoception. There's an awareness of what's happening with the body, heart, soul, and mind in relationship to life and other people. There's an ability to live life and not just solely mind.

What often keeps you distant from another person includes criticism, fear of criticism, comparisons, unhealed shame, limited thinking from unexamined beliefs, betrayals, lack of trust, abandonment, past rejection, unworthiness, entitlement, all the stuff of the terrified, victim self. Various combinations of these lived experiences keep you disconnected from the arena of your soul, locked outside the domain of your vulnerability, your failures, emotional bruises, and the humanity that we share. With protected, cloaked hearts, you can remain at a distance from other people in all those places and spaces.

What brings you emotionally closer to other people continues to be vulnerability, honesty, and courage. You must feel safe enough and brave enough to break through the hard shell you've likely created around your heart. In grief and love, you are part of the interconnected web of existence. Maybe you came here to hold compassionate space for hurts, failings, foibles of your own and other people's and to celebrate the gifts, strengths, and skills within yourself and other individuals. Maybe, like me, you came here to love and be loved in return.

May you experience emotional closeness with those you love. May you know the experience of being valued by another human being no matter your flaws, failings, or foibles. May you become the person that your heart knows you are.

At the Core

Compassion in the guts
In the pelvis
The womb of it all,
Where empathy merges
With walking shoes
Boots
Sandals or
Bare feet.
Feeling the earth
Of real life lived
Through another's experience
Which you feel as your own
In the whole
Of you.

Courage in
The heart
To flow emotion
As
Energy in motion.

Brave enough
To break your
Heart wide open
And grieve in
The middle
Of a room
On knees, shaking,
Wailing, rocking,
Sobbing
Streaming.
Pouring down
A cascade of
Unleashed salt waters
Escaping through
Every cavernous
passageway
Rhythmic and
Cleansing.

Brave enough to
Roll on the floor
Stomach muscles flexing
Contracting
Labia laughing
Mouth wide open
Lilting, vibrating
Soft tongue resting, nestling
Pulsing
Rippling waves

Of
Releasing.

Brave enough
To surrender
And let go
Multiple orgasms
Of Belly Laughing
Bravery.

Love in your
Throat
Chest
Voice box
Singing the song
Of your
Completeness
A circle of
Rainbow words
Flowing, swirling
Babbling joyfully
Like bubbles blown from
Liquid soap,
Dripping from a
Pink magic wand.
Free to speak love,
Sing love
See love from the
Inside of

Vocal chords
Interwoven and soothed by
Grace and Forgiveness.

Clear,
Aligned
Planking strong
Even in the
Surrender to the floor
Hold the world.
Stretch high.
Dignity, strength
Firm in the core
Of who You Are.

Beauty Truth Love=You

He ruptured your hymen; he didn't break you.
You are more than that moment of
Piercing pain, gasping for breath,
Yelling, "Do you feel better now?"
Like he relieved himself inside you
Rather than uplift and glorify you.

You struggled to push him far away.
You weren't strong enough
To break the grasp of
Hands on your wrists.
Now your strength resides
Inside your faith,
Your courage, and your grace.

His manhood cannot
Reach you for you
Dwell in the crevices
Of creative power and
In a womb of possibilities.

Your Mighty
Kindness, Compassion,
Resilience
Self-Love and Self-Worth
Burn bright.

Discernment, deep equanimity
Join as the dual guides
To an Enduring trust
An unrelenting will to thrive.

Your voice rings loud, clear, and bold.
You speak from the depths of your truth
Passionate to relish
Your body vessel as
A goddess with breadth, depth, width, height
Muscle, mass, hips, lips, breasts, eyes
Sparkling
A thousand moments of dignity
Waking up and walking tall.

Seeds unleashed grow flowers
Blooming gloriously in your heart.
Your beauty radiates each day
In colorful hues and highlights.
Streaks and shrieks of light and laughter.

Living a wholehearted life
With sweetness after that bitter
Becomes your greatest revenge.

You are exuberantly alive
Free
A force of love
In our world.

Swim

Plunge into the icy blue.
Stretch whole body long,
Feet flutter
Underwater.

Arms create the
S cross top,
Pulling
Hands like paddles.

Rhythmic breaths,
Blowing bubbles
That tickle the belly.

A Black Line
Guiding
Rolling head up through
Skimming, rolling waves.

Bright yellow, blue lane
Dividers containing

Your race,
Your progress.

Boundaries allow
Freedom, move
At your pace.

Not knowing
Or seeing what anyone
Else is doing or being.

Who are you in your
Lane as the world
Changes,
Lives end,
Lungs collapse?

Can you keep moving in
A pool of
Despair without
Being swallowed
Whole?
Accept the
Depth of darkness.
Breech the surface
Of abandonment.
Inhale
Fresh perspectives.

Exhale
Hostage held truths.

The wall of awe
Awaits
At a distance.

Swim like
Lives
Depend on
The wake
That love
Passion
Create.

To Be Chosen

I remember being in elementary school out on the playground.

"Red Rover. Red Rover. Send Sally right over!"

I tightly clasped the hands of the children on either side of me. The three of us would not be the ones who let Sally break our sealed bond. We refused to be the "weak link" in the long line of children chanting.

What a horrible game this was for me. Did any child ever really want to be chosen to run through the clasped hands of classmates? For me, it felt like that familiar rock in a hard place wanting your name called out because that meant the kids knew you existed and not ever wanting your name called out because you'd fail. Oh, that awful scared feeling of anticipated public humiliation if you weren't big enough or fast enough to burst through those seemingly bonded with glue hands. And then the laughter would come that inevitably occurred when a child did not break through the line of the opposite team. Ugh.

I've forgotten what happened in the game to the child after she failed her teammates. I viscerally remember more tormenting, jeering, and laughing. Then the seemingly enduring public shame of not ever having your name called, having your name called last, when teams got formed. The rejection of certain classmates and me at recess during the game of "red rover" left us in that place of pseudo-invisibility, yet painfully visible for our "unwanted" status because the adults on the playground would insist that the game include everyone.

In a different scenario, when I was ten years old, I managed to swim swiftly during summer swim team season and won trophies, including the most valuable girl swimmer trophy. I could hardly take in this moment of "being chosen." The cheering teammates, coaches, parents standing up, wildly applauding, completely overwhelmed me. The humiliation of all my other mistakes or perceived by others' failings burned too fiercely. Plus, I anticipated demeaning, twisted comments when I returned to my parent's house. "Getting a big head" was an anathema.

My heart pounded with fear. I wanted to sink into the floor and hand the trophy to at least ten other deserving teammates. My face burned with embarrassment while my stomach did uncontrollable somersaults. I prayed I wouldn't throw up. This type of "being chosen" felt like a shame storm swirling around a so-called happy moment, what another child might experience as a joyous occasion. What I believed about myself, what I had been told repeatedly by specific adults, did not translate into "most valuable" anything.

Years later, I discovered these trophies in a box. While my infant son napped, my pre-school-aged daughter and I explored some cabinets. I pulled out the statues. Taken by the shine, the shape of the bent-over woman bodies clad in metal suits and caps in that ready to dive posture, my daughter asked if she could hold them. I said, "Of course. They've just been sitting in a box." Her small hands tenderly held the trophies. She began playing with them on the floor, bringing each one to life by talking out loud, giving them voices. She uttered kind words as these shiny metal bodies on those wood platforms flowed through the air guided by her hands and arms. My daughter played like children enjoy a tea party with their stuffed animals and dolls.

As I watched her, I felt deep humiliation. I had imbued these awards with the private put-downs, the cruel shaming sessions I had endured. At this juncture, I had begun learning about the wisdom of feng shui, so I knew belongings came with positive stories, associations, memories, or negative ones. I realized that I had to dispose of these trophies to rid myself of the negative energy.

After she completed her play, we placed them back in the box. Later that day, I carried the box of trophies to the large green trash container behind the garage. My need for relief outweighed everything else. I trusted that letting go of those trophies would help me continue to untangle my inner world of the awful feelings and memories that still hurt deeply.

Now, my more healed, wiser, more dignified self can, in my mind's eye, gently hold the hand of my 10-year-old self to assure her that she can allow the jubilation and love from all those cheering parents, teammates, and coaches into her heart. Being able to receive love graciously along with the joyful energy of being chosen and celebrated continues to be brave, sometimes uncomfortable, yet healing and transformative work for me.

Unblocking the heart to let go of the shame steeped words that become internal beliefs and choosing to celebrate your actual accomplishments, distinctions, and awards can be a courageous walk for those of us who've felt undeserving in any way. It's the opposite affliction of those who feel entitled to every award and swagger with bragging. Somewhere in the middle place remains the choice of one's inner dignity and humility regardless of external rewards or reactions of other people.

Have you bravely chosen the qualities of your character? Are you continuing to cultivate an enduring sense of inner dignity, worth, and humility that no words or awards can touch? Have you chosen your perfectly imperfect self, your essential self?

Being accepted for all that you are: your expressions, skills, capacities, learnings which include your goodness, kindness, bursts of joy, meltdowns, frustrations, fears, terrors, mistakes, accomplishments, awards, resilience, courage, intelligence, silliness, and sass; compassion for your humanity emerges. You can choose to deeply accept yourself even though you might still feel a bit tender from too many years of the bruising ache of non-acceptance by people with whom you had desperately yearned to be accepted and celebrated. Rather than endlessly waiting for what other people may never be able to do, you can choose yourself.

Radical acceptance, the capacity to choose whatever life

brings, frees you to summon inner strength. Knowing you have gained skills, demonstrated courage, you can nourish an enduring inner dignity, a deep acceptance of yourself. Life will continue to deliver experiences that are uncomfortable or challenging no matter your preferences. That's the design of life. Choosing life as it is in this moment becomes a pathway to freedom and peace.

May you tenderly clasp your own hands in a beautiful bond of acceptance. May you hold your sweet face gently in both your hands with love, choosing fully to embrace your perfectly imperfect self. May you choose to see your whole self through eyes of compassion and grace.

Paper Mache

Words spoken
From the heart
Once deflected,
Captured
Twisted, repurposed
Into piercing weapons
Boomerang
Slicing.

Syrupy sweet
Words
From others
Seem
Hopeful.
Mouth
Watering,
Poured,
Pooling,
Seductive.
A fleeting
Promise

Turning
Too quickly
To Dark
Tongue
Dirt spittle.

Like
A beautiful
Colorfully
Wrapped
Crinkling
Candy that
Tastes
Horehound
Bitter in your
Mouth.

Politely
Acknowledge
Kind words
At a Far
Distance.

Unaware how
Thick the
Cast
Formed
Around

A tender
Chest.

In safety
Unwind.
Crack open
White
Paper Mache.

Resonant
Meaningful
Radiant
Genuine
Loving
Words
Softly sink
Into an
Exposed
Heaving
Warmed
Glowing
Opened
Heart.

Princess's Soft Singing

$\mathcal{G}$rowing up surrounded by tortured, unpredictable adults, you listen to her whispers in natural places of trust that mirror all tender parts of yourself you must keep hidden from the outer world of cacophony, chaos, and cruelty. She invites you.

"Pretend a wonderful fairy tale, Prince Charming shapeshifting into your beautiful Princess Self. Your still small voice. She's the goddess inside of you! She loves you, protects you. She knows you will live, grow, flourish."

Your courageous princess's soft singing comforts you from deep inside a rapidly beating heart. You listen closely to her lullabies over days, nightmares, months, seasons, decades. Connecting with the core of her being and your strong runner's legs, you burst forth into a soul haven aligned with fearless radiance and the grace of joyful laughter.

"Live here!" she declares. "Thrive in this place. Live your dreams awake! You are me, and I have always been You!"

Sweeping Strokes

Here in the dark, inky-dot places, she can begin to notice lighter hues of blue-like the skies she sees outside of gloomy buildings filled with grumpy people. Out of the inkblots whooshes the uplift of space, a breathing room of clouds-white, puffy, lighthearted, swirling, shapeshifting, dancing in the atmosphere where birds soar free.

Wild geese, ducks, herons know when to open their wings.

She lies down to sleep; inhale, one, two, three, four. Hold breath. One, two, three, four. Exhale, one, two, three, four, hold breath. One, two, three, four, inhale, hold breath. This pattern repeats while drifting into a dream-filled sleep with both ghosts, goddesses guiding her back to the murky, dark depths of past mud-puddle days that seemed to last forever. Her heart falls beneath the shallow waters of leaves, autumn leaves of reds, rust, and gold flowing on the surface. Underneath the shallows remain nuggets of discovery, of truths unexpressed, yearning to be spoken. Why, when, how dare you-s. The what's wrong with me hurts, haunted wounds, unwilling to dislodge themselves from the sides of a cavernous cave.

Hold on to the breath. Let go of the depth of soul-wrenching loss of what others claim can be a carefree childhood. Chasing butterflies, digging in the dirt, getting black soil caught under fingernails from plunging two tiny hands into the layers of crumbled, caked-on dirt where seeds go, where bugs go, where more flat rocks reveal themselves. How deep can she swim in the dark depths, searching for a tiny girl body soiled at the evil doings of a tortured being? Taking long, sweeping strokes back up to the surface, she pulls forward the truth of light. No action done to a tiny body can ever spoil her spirit, her soul of light, the woman, goddess of radiance she becomes in the creamy, delicious places of divine safety, faithful generosity.

Beauty Pageant Drop-Out

Slopping wet clay globs of make-up on my face and neck, standing in front of a group of people oblivious to me, I awoke, remembering the time my mother insisted I enter a beauty pageant.

"It's for a *scholarship*!" she insisted.

While the word "scholarship" indeed came in the event title, this was a beauty pageant. All the contestants would don a swimsuit, present a talent, and answer "World Peace" to the question, "What is your highest aspiration?" This competition was not Jeopardy or Lego robotics.

Because I stood only 5'3" the organizers directed me to the children's section to select two outfits for a fashion show luncheon that would take place a couple of months before the pageant. As a high school junior, I painfully knew each body flaw I possessed; like hot flaming shame characters doing their best to berate me.

My comfort zone centered on books and classrooms, not racks of clothing. Academically, I excelled; socially, I struggled to fit in. Too many times popular girls made fun of me. Yet, when one of them would encounter me alone in the bathroom washing our hands at the sink together, she'd be kind, even admiring of me. I concluded-girls alone, kind; girls in a group-mean.

One day at a restroom sink encounter, one of the popular girls handed me an envelope with my name scribbled on the front. As I gently tugged on the inside decorative card "It's a Party" leapt out at me.

Astonished, I happily accepted the invitation to a slumber party which included cheerleaders and beautiful girls who dated the handsome, intelligent, and athletic guys. In my naivete, I thought I had been accepted into their cherished ranks.

Playing games in our pajamas, some girls squealed that all our bras had been put in the freezer. That quickly turned out to be a lie. My bra had been selected as the solo cold "prize."

One girl grabbed my bra and swung it around the kitchen while the rest of the girls laughed and pointed at me. Red-faced and nauseous, I walked to the bathroom and puked into the toilet. I don't remember packing up my things or calling my dad to come get me.

I do remember standing patiently at the curb with my overnight backpack hung with a rolled-up sleeping bag waiting for our family's blue Chevy station wagon. The dark night, the rustling of leaves on the trees welcomed me as they always had. Taking in big gulps of air, I felt the nausea dissipate as tears slid down my face, first warm then turning cold as the night autumn air met my hot sadness.

How would I ever face any of those girls during the next week of school?

Sitting in a chair as a woman put make-up on my face before the fashion show luncheon, I cringed. Another woman, who had already been critical of my thighs, walked over. She pronounced, "If she has those ugly blemishes on Pageant Night, be certain to use this product on her face as it will cover those unsightly pimples." Officially I felt like a permanently flawed object, a walking blemish, a disgrace.

How I sauntered through that room in the manner the director had taught us, while wearing a floral print sleeveless dress and then a matching lime green terry cloth shorts & top with sandals, I do not know. I barely smiled. When I did smile, my mouth remained shut tight; a pressed-lipped, fake face on top of a growing fury that likely flashed in my eyes. The faces of the grown women sitting at their white-clothed draped round tables became a blur. I focused on the side walls of the hotel banquet room during these modeling struts of objectification. I can still hear the woman on the microphone, "This sporty outfit will eventually look amazing after Laura has a summertime tan and trim thighs."

Afterward, while riding in the backseat of the car with my mother driving, I made my fierce declaration to my mother:

"I quit! I refuse to be in this pageant! I hate this! The women are mean! I don't care about the scholarship money! I'm hideous looking, and I will not win!"

A fiery argument with my mother erupted in the car.

Back at my parent's house, my dad offered the backup I needed. As I sat at the top of the stairs, I overheard my dad speak after my mother's tirade. *I believe it's important to honor*

Laura's choice. If she doesn't want to compete in this pageant, then I say she doesn't compete in the pageant."

Beauty pageant drop-out got added to my life experiences resume.

Years later after divorcing my second husband, who had made certain I knew I did not have a large enough bust or butt throughout our 22 years of marriage, I finally discarded my body dysmorphia. I set free most of the shamefear inside of me.

My daughter appreciated me for not shaming her body as she observed her female college friends struggling with poor body image. I realized at that moment that I had broken the cycle with my daughter. When I birthed her, I remembered vowing not to dump that dysfunctional energy into her reality. I focused my attention on her interests, what brought her joy in being alive, her courage, resilience in facing challenges, healthy eating, and activity. I had focused on healing my patterns in conversations with other people instead of speaking in front of her.

Being vibrantly healthy in mind, heart, body, and soul became more important than external packaging. How people treat other people continues to be where I pay close attention. A person's packaging may look all polished, but those inner character qualities matter most of all. Cultivating an internal radiance of dignity, compassion, kindness, courage, intellectual humility carries lifelong credibility.

Some people did not arrive on the planet to be eye candy or bullies. Some people are here to create, to express themselves, to break free from ancestral patterns, to defy worn-out paradigms, and live true to their soul's callings.

An obsessive focus on external beauty can distract you from passionate, purposeful pursuits.

Have you learned to be kind to yourself no matter what you look like?

May you unlearn the legacy of body shame and shift your life energy to creative pursuits that bring you joy. May you realize that from the moment you were born you were a beautiful soul with unique gifts to be generously shared with our world.

Volitional

You can't make me!
I can choose!
It's My life not your
Suffocating Expectations.
Access Denied to
My Inner World.
You can
Spit cruel words.
Rage like you
Want me to die.
I am rising Inside
And there's nothing
You can do about that!
My brain is mine.
My heart is mine.
My bones and lustful
Feelings are mine.
Words that bubble
Up from the bowels of me
Tongue, lining of lips,
Breasts, hips

Mine.
You can lock me in
A room.
Songs sing inside
Memories,
Imagination,
Sweat,
Breath,
Lungs, ribs
Vulva
A womb that grew
Two babies.
All mine.

Positive gratitude
Cannot manipulate God
To Grant
Three-Year-Old
Gimmee Game
Of Demands, wants,
Aspirations, desires,
Wishes, dreams, or hopes.

Accept exactly the Way Life
Is.
People, inanimate
Objects work or not.
Cuss at the
Computer that

Doesn't stop beeping,
People who
Choose differently
than you.
OR
Practice softening
Sphincter
Every single time
Underwear gets in a wad like
A wedgie, tangled thong.
Choose wispy hair.
Choose pandemic.
Choose kindness.
Choose this moment.
Right Here.
Right Now.

Shadows

Bask in the sunshine,
Gently notice your shadow.

Bright full moonlight
Creates another image.

A silhouette like silence moves,
Stands still,
Dances,
A forever quiet partner,
Bearing witness to the
Unspoken
Unspeakable
Unbroken
Hidden eclipse.

What blocks your view of vast possibilities,
Enduring love?

What causes you to hide from your
Beautiful self?

Night
Mares gallop
Into your sweat soaked
Bed,
Guide you to confront truths
You've given up to the darkness.

What remains in the underbelly
Whispers to be valued,
Seen through a beam of grace.

When the sunshine shadows and
Moon shadows finally embrace, a
New day dawns at dusk.

The birthing of your soul begins.

Bearing Witness

After all these years
You finally share realizations,
Your heartfelt apologies
For what you did, said.

You recognize their love
For each other often exceeded
And excluded us.

You appreciate that
As an adult perhaps you possessed
Skills to navigate her cruel words,
Deeds that I did not
as a child inside the
Oak Hill House.

After all these years
You wrote that you see,
Hear,
Value me.

You celebrate the
Voice I found, the happiness,
Love I live.

You awakened and
Opened your eyes.
Compassion, kindness,
Love matter the most.

As the sole courageous one
To step forward after
All these years, please
Know how grateful I am
To be fully vindicated,
Affirmed.

Birthed from a darkened womb of denial,
Raw, real truths
Grow.

Run free with
Strong muscular legs
Around deep waters of peace.
You and I can
Embrace in the radiant light
Of mutual awareness
After all these years.

Blooming Lotus Flower

After I became single, I dated a man I met business networking. I learned a great deal about myself during this short period as I brought an end to my pattern of being connected to people who struggled to bring their best selves to the table with me. During our entire time together, I grew my "witness consciousness," that part of me who watches my behaviors, words, feelings, body sensations and observes what others say and do.

I remember many moments during our time together when I internally threw a "flag on the play" as I witnessed unkind behaviors. I discovered people voice their insecurities in different ways, and some deliver sarcasm liberally. The insecure voices in my head became much quieter. The work to make peace internally remained mine to do.

On one occasion, at an open networking event, I walked up to a woman to introduce myself and learn what she did. When she asked me about my company, Cherish Your World, I began to share how I help people and why I'm passionate about the principles and practices of feng shui. The man I was dating approached us, looked at the woman, and said, laughing, "Don't listen to her. She doesn't know what she's talking about!"

The woman looked at him, said something to him that I don't remember, and returned to our conversation. I remember thinking that he wasn't funny, nor was his comment kind or supportive. Some part of me felt foolish, small, and diminished, the way I had felt many times in my life.

As his birthday approached, I became inspired, and a fun idea bubbled up. Instead of purchasing a gift, I chose to create a collage for him of many things he loved from his childhood and life. When I joined him and his friends at a fancy restaurant to celebrate, I handed him the collage. He looked at me and said, laughing, "Wow. You have too much time on your hands!"

I remained silent. His close friend, who witnessed his response, approached me, and said, "That was a kind, thoughtful gift you created for him."

Again, I watched as most of me bore witness to his demeanor, words, and deeds. A part of me shrank into small, foolish embarrassment. Another part of me, a stronger, more confident me, knew he had revealed himself, once again, and that I no longer needed to collect evidence of the not good fit we were as a couple. In many ways we remain very different people. I chose to stay at the restaurant and quietly observe him with his close friends as they drank and ate. Like an anthropologist, I silently ate my meal in quiet discomfort mixed with gratitude.

A few weeks later, I ended our dating experience together. The small, foolish, embarrassed part of me had shrunk. The courageous, confident, worthy part of me had expanded. I grieved as I noticed a whole other part of me had fallen in love with this gentleman, for he is a good man, just not a right fit for me. I had experienced a full array of his expressions without any agenda to alter who he was. I had observed my responses and what had come alive inside of me during our time together. These realizations live to this day as my breakthroughs.

I'm grateful for every single moment because this experience became a place in which to leap forward with greater clarity about who I wanted to become, the ways I am fortunate to love and honor myself and other people.

This year I have decided to create a collage of all the things I love about my life. I have created collages for several other people I love and have not yet made one for me. I have spent a lifetime bearing witness to other people in their humanity and their greatness, their flaws, and fabulousness. I believe the time to take ownership of my voice, multifaceted expressions, and passions is now.

As a gift of integration to a world of people who've held up mirrors to my goodness that I have, at times, deflected, I no longer have to shrink from the truths of who I am, what I came here to share, why I'm on the planet. I can fully bloom like a lotus flower growing from the mud.

When I observe other people from that silent, non-judgmental space inside, I learn a wealth of information that leads to greater understanding from an expansive, compassionate place. People show me who they are with their words and deeds. I reveal myself through my words, deeds, or silence.

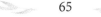

When I pay attention from my heart, I notice a great deal about friends, strangers, colleagues, acquaintances, companions, clients, children, and family. Listening beyond my ears or busy mind while dropping into my loving, quiet witness, I can see through eyes of awareness and discernment. I make better choices when I dispassionately collect information about myself and other people through the lens of my dignity, vulnerability, and value. The people I walk towards and choose to be with for a reason, a season, or a lifetime often reveals what I most need to learn about myself, about being a patient, loving, self-aware adult person.

May you grow in self-awareness as you integrate all the pieces and parts of yourself. May you come to know your true, beautiful self. May you see yourself through the eyes and hearts of those who truly cherish you because they have learned to love themselves.

QUIRKY

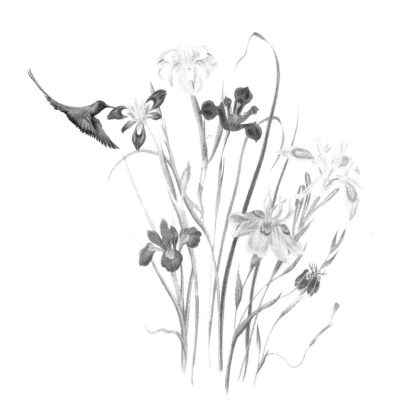

Human Exoskeleton

Vacated long ago
Broken down structure
A reminder the
Past existed.

Unmaintained
Alone
Forlorn
Unloved
Abandoned on the
Street.

Empty of human life,
Sounds, steps,
Voices, energy,
Industry.

Were you loved
At the
Ribbon cutting?

The doors opening
Grand and wide?

Who forgot you?
Who declared you
Unworthy of
Repair
Remodel
Tender love,
Care?

Cheaper to leave
You to the dirt.
Too expensive.
Misguided allocation of
Resources.
A cascade of
Choices where you
Got the short stick.

Did they paint
You vibrant before or
After you crumbled,
Lost your head and
Guts?

A colorful
Façade reminder
Of the

Glory days
Or an attempt
To brighten
The sore eye
You now are.

How long will
You languish as this
Human exoskeleton?
At what moment will
All your remaining
Exterior crash to
The ground
Or be worn away
By rain, sleet, snow,
Winds of time?

I see your
Decrepit
Loneliness,
A shell of what
You were.
Humans fled
Far, far
Away.

I wish
You gentle hospice
Care from

Nature's mother
Who will forever
Hold you in
Grace
From dusk
To dust.

What Are the Contents of Your Character?

Here are some of mine:

98 pounds of perseverance
5 gallons courage
20 gigabytes compassion
2 Tbsp. embarrassment
1 degree Fahrenheit self-pity
3/4 cups shame
5 years sass
1/2 tsp. annoyance
6 degrees Grrrrrr!
A galaxy of Love
½ tsp. resentment
1 mile I don't wanna!
2 Tbsp. you're not gonna make me!
40,000 hours creativity
40 megabytes resilience
Exponential energy
80000 pints hilarious laughter
20 tons gratitude
15 lbs. imagination

11 quarts vision

5 liters optimism

9 decades self-discovery

1,111 past lives

5 x 9 + (200 − 7) x 538 yards of humility

200 dark chocolate bars of tenderness

50 lbs. fly on the wall/inner observer

2 Truckloads of tenderness

100 mph of curiosity

Copious cups of contentment

Gobs of grace

$\mathcal{M}$ix with 128 kilograms of kindness. Boil with 8 pounds of passion. Bake in the warmth of the sun. Cool in the moonlit, star-filled sky. Slice with care. Serve with a dollop of daydreaming. Deliver with full responsibility. Makes enough to inspire many.

Characters Chattering

*F*eng shui invites us to look and listen with our open eyes and ears. What are your belongings showing or telling you about your life? What are those voices, maybe entire characters, inside of you saying and feeling? Do those thoughts and feelings support your life purpose, your joy in living? How old or young are those "voices"?

With much joy, I've lately been naming the "thoughts/feelings" inside of me to see who has grabbed a hold of the talking stick, that conch shell, or the microphone in my lively internal sixth grade or kindergarten classroom-depending on the day. Is Pity Party Patty whining because she's been comparing her life to the stunningly smart, productive, and beautiful other girls? Has Annoyed Andrea managed to get her underwear in a bunch because the soap dispenser clogged again? Did a torrent of dad memories wash over Grieving Greta? Then her cell phone pings and Concerned Caring Cora quickly texts back a supportive, loving reply to a friend having a rough day. Still in the back of the room Unworthy Ursula persists in throwing wet, hot, shame towels which flop onto the floor failing to stifle every single sparkling idea that bursts out of Inspired Ivy. Then Analytical Slightly Anxious Anna timidly steps up to a flip chart with several colorful Sharpies to create a ridiculous looking spreadsheet, flow chart, or spider web map attempting to reign in these middle school kindergartners into a sane explanation of an obvious, not obvious recent triggering incident that stirred everyone up into a frenzy.

You are probably wondering how the heck I ever get anything accomplished. I often wonder about this, too. I believe that my Disciplined Doreen regularly takes charge of all these other parts of me by walking into the room and saying firmly with utter clarity, "Guys, we have to get some sh&* done today. I hear you and feel you, but life is NOW. I promise to listen to you with rapt attention tomorrow morning when we are running around the lake. You can tell me all your ideas, cry tears of sadness, and bitch about what has you experiencing that wedgie! We'll also get a chance to hear the geese and ducks, feel the cold air, and breathe rhythmically. I love you all so much, but seriously, I get to compose a newsletter blog thing."

Our physical belongings are blathering their joys and laments, too, like all the toys from the Toy Story movies. If you haven't seen the Toy Story movies, I highly recommend them for the heartwarming feng shui wisdom offered. Gosh, just when you thought your life couldn't get any noisier. And by now, I'm certain you've noticed that I haven't even layered in the sound of the furnace blowing, the pings of technology, the paper airplanes wafting through the air, the bubble gum popping.

Meditation, mindfulness, and yoga practice have taught me the benefits of returning many times to a centered place of deep quiet inside me. Taking deep, slow breaths, feeling my body sensations, the fuzzy socks on my feet, observing where my tongue is inside of my mouth, looking around at beautiful objects in the room, and out the windows at the gorgeous sky and trees. If there's not a fire in the kitchen or my dog placing her nose on my leg cueing me to take her out for that bio break, I ask myself, "What would Loving Laura do now? or Worthy Wendy?" These are two of my all-time favorite characters who regularly hold hands with Hilarious Heloise, Compassionate Caroline, Kind Karen, and Courageous Catalina.

At the end of the day, Present Precious brings them all together in the room to sit down on a rug. She beams a silent light of enduring, unshakeable love and gratitude and gives them all warm hugs. Aren't you relieved that you aren't my Sweet Love? Ah, the earful he receives while on a date with all of us. LOL. Wow. Ah, what an exceptional man.

May you listen and embrace all the parts of your Self with enduring love and gratitude. May you discover the joy of intermittent quiet in a noisy world. May you laugh at all your inner characters unless you don't have any-in that case you can laugh at mine because maybe I'm the only one-oh gosh I hope not-who richly entertains herself with no one in the room!

Priscilla, Panties in a Wad

Irritated,
Annoyed,
Critical,
Prickly, Prissy,
Cranky
Part of me.
Thought
She had to be
Perfect,
That life
Would be
Kind always, especially
If she behaved,
Performed, perfected,
Followed the rules.
The sun shines brightly
On this balmy December day
After many days of frosty,
Biting, wind chills.
In the peacefulness of the
Carolina Blue sky, a deeper

Truth reveals itself.
Life is life
At the source is
Love.
Here all is radiant.
Even inside a dark well
Covered over by burrs, nettles, branches,
And bruised on the ground prickly pears. Soft,
Tender, juicy inside are you, my sweet
Priscilla.
I love you in your
Itchy, scratchiness for
You just want peace.
A slice of quiet solitude nestled
Next to the soft white clouds
Drifting asleep, awake,
Commando.

Forgive Your Self

Such important work for a human being—
To feel regret,
Remorse,
To experience deeply, broadly the
Impact
Words, deeds have on other people.
Staring in the mirror right at a shamefear face.
No longer stuffing these feelings
In a dusty box on top of a shelf,
In the corner of an attic,
A moldy crate in a
Damp creepy basement, or
Inside the lining of arteries,
Running away from the most
Important muscle.
Forgiving self can be
Immeasurably more difficult
Then forgiving cruel words, deeds of others,
The silent complicity of indifferent ones.
Attached to
Nice Girl

Kind Girl
Sweet Girl
Quiet Girl
Silent Girl
Invisible Girl
To Look at *Ugh*
Mean Girl
Jealous Girl
Resentful Girl
Salty Sailor Mouth Girl
Cornered Animal Spitting Nails Fierce Girl
Judgmental Girl
Ugh

Inner Quiet One
Watches scenes
Of younger hurting
Warriors
Using eyes of
Understanding
Compassion.

That's what
Unresolved trauma
Looks like.

Wounded ones
Become fiery fighters
Sometimes

Out of their minds,
Hurting others and
Themselves
Until those paths
Become bankrupt.

Choose healthy ways
To purge the pain
Kick boxing
Martial Arts
NIA Dance
Yoga Flow
Running, swimming, dancing
Bawling, sobbing, crying
MOVE the BODY!
Scream F*CK F*CK F*CK
To the breezes.
Carry wild words
Into
Rumbling, crackling
Thunderstorms.

Forgive self.
A practice like
Cleaning a house.
A cycle, a rhythm.
Keep purging
All that Past.
All of It.

Feeling Remorse
Is the Price of
Freedom in
Heart &
Being.

Out of Pocket, Powered Up

This morning I woke up to a black screen on my cell phone. I noticed yesterday that the power had declined rapidly even after starting the day at 100 percent. Two weeks ago, I had replaced cords that had gone bad. I knew that wasn't the issue. I sought wisdom from my in-house tech person. How fortunate I am that this person is my SL (Sweet Love).

"Hey, hon, my phone isn't holding a charge."

"Your phone battery needs to be replaced."

"Oh, okay. I'll take care of this today."

I felt too embarrassed to admit that I didn't know that cell phones come with batteries. I knew that the smoke detectors hold those Energizer Bunny guys inside with plastic grips that sometimes make it impossible to replace with the metal Lego-like brick ones. I wondered if some angry person in another country intentionally zapped my phone with some software virus called Cootie Chocolate Cookie. This would be distinct from Cootie Covid19, which sadly has caused sickness, pandemonium, global pandemic, deaths, countless challenges. I quickly shifted my thoughts. *I have a first-world issue. I'll be inconvenienced for a few hours. I'm dipping my big toe in a modified "off the grid" reality. How addicted might I be to this "I have my life stored in this thing!" device?*

After handling several tasks for a client, I drove to Best Buy, donned my mask, and waited to speak to a man behind the Geek Squad counter. I explained my predicament. He asked if I had backed up my cell phone. Not wanting to appear ignorant, I said,

"Uh, I think so."

I know what a backed-up sink looks like, what a backed-up toilet smells like, and what a backed-up digestive tract feels like. I have even experienced a basement sewage backup. *How was I supposed to know about the clogged passageways in a cell phone? Oh, right!! Back up in the tech world means Save, Save, Save-have a plan B, C, D, and E!! Ah, the language thing, again. Ack!*

So, this is like my paper calendar, pens, and paper journals? I have this kind of "backup" system with my Boom Box-thank goodness-along with actual Compact Discs I can play to hear music since my cell phone is dead and won't stream Barbra Streisand Radio through Spotify. Thank goodness for my Back-Up Belongings!

"Ma'am."

The man behind the counter startled me back to the moment.

I handed him my phone after entering in my password.

He swiftly tapped to all the right places on the phone like the amazing being he indeed is.

"You have not backed up your phone. You need to do this first. You need to save things to iCloud, especially photographs. I can schedule your battery replacement for two days from now. Keep in mind that when the battery is removed it might break this other thing in your phone and your whole phone will need to be replaced. Apple will replace your phone if that happens."

Wait, WHAT? How much will this cost me? Are you serious?! Replacing the battery may mean my entire phone could be replaced---that I might lose everything that's stored in the phone?!? WTF?! I thought clouds were white puffy formations of what will become precipitation coming down from the sky--- cumulus, cirrus, nimbostratus, cumulonimbus. Clearly, I know much more about clouds in the sky than I do about iCloud. I wonder if you, young man, know all the types of clouds. Actually, yeah, you probably do. Sigh.

I calmly looked at the getting younger by the minute, man, and said, "Yes, I will save things to the clouds and can schedule for your first opening on Thursday. Thank you so much, Sir."

When I arrived home, I did the steps he showed me in hopes that I saved the cell phone content which I have come to rely on.

At hour six of no cell phone, I managed to go on a run in the cold, brisk air and sunshine at the lake, shower, dress, eat breakfast, meditate, listen to an entire CD on my Boom Box, type this essay, hug, and kiss my Sweet Love, hang up damp, clean running gear on my dry rack, drink water, look at the Carolina blue sky and all the almost bare trees, and feel immense appreciation for the challenge of today. My panties have not gotten bunched up or in a wad. I get to drive to meet my poet friends outside in the sunshine in our coats and masks to read poetry to one another, to stand at the intersection with a Love sign, wave, and smile at all my neighbors driving or walking by with joy in my heart.

I get to power up a human heart battery with activities that keep me connected to Mother Earth, people I love who love me. And I took a few moments to write a long letter of gratitude to my cell phone for I realize that small computer I hold in my hand frees me to be in a larger world of people, photographs, texts, heartfelt conversations of loving kindness and laughter, Facebook posts---all pathways to share love, humor, rapture for this beautiful, most precious life. From my heart and mind, I get to create, savor, and live connected with all people who can see those gorgeous cumulus clouds in the sky on a bright sunny day.

May you choose consciously, purposefully to stay connected to who and what inspires you to be all in for this one and only wondrous life you get to live.

Lost

Where are you?

Listening with
Rapt attention,
Waiting to hear
The next
Throaty, choked back,
Hacked up
Syllable.

A
Phrase now blathering
From searching
Toes that
Felt the insides of too
Many
Hand-me-Down
Buster Browns.

Where are the
Brave clogs that fit

Your sweet feet?
Your feet that have
Wandered for years
In other people's
Too roomy, too tight,
Too shiny,
Ridiculously Not *you*
Shoes.

Desperately
Yearning for
Meaningful
Understanding,
Connection,
To
What seems forever
Lost.

Not ever
Found in
That empty closet
Stuffed with
Distracting detritus from
Impossible
Dreams.

Where are you?

For You

Grown Up
Professional

Quite a shift
From the other
Ones, low
Riders,
Not Sexy
Or fun.

Daughter
First sees you
Had no
Idea you'd
Make me
Feel
Strong,
Empowered.

Security check
Point at Court.

I cannot curl my
Toes.
I'm a
Petrified Plaintiff
Petitioning for
Freedom.

Down the long
Sterile hospital hallway,
Glaring florescent lights
To see my son.
Too many times.
He lives.

Home again,
I weep
While curled
In a ball
Next to you.

Networking.
Held me tall,
Proud. Right leg
Quivers uncontrollably
First, of many
Elevator speeches.

Grounding in
Joy,

Heart connection.
A handsome,
Self-aware, sweet
Love. On my feet,
Standing when
He kisses me the
First time.

Packing excitedly.
Lovingly
Bound
For soul home of
Mountains,
Another first.

Upright
In autumn
Sunshine
At an intersection.
Joyfully smiling, waving.
Choose
Love for Love.

Brought me
To this day,
This moment
Of knowing.
Not certain
I could be

Here without you.
Patiently
Waiting for
Another adventure.
Grateful, for you,
My Brave Boots.

Cutting the Rope

Between
Known
Unknown.
What I don't know
That I don't know
About me,
People,
Life.

Disorienting.
Quicksand.
No sea legs
Or hand to hold
Onto for
Dear Life.

On a rock climb
Away from clenching to
Those who wish you
Death.

Courageously
Cutting the rope.
Saving the one
Life You
Could
Save.

Out of Touch 2020

Experiencing a certain
Life on the edge.
Living at an extreme
Of little or no touch.

No hugs, handshakes
Gentle, warm hand, fingers intertwining
With our own.

No Skin warming skin,
Soft palms holding our faces.

Now
Eyes peering into eyes,
At a distance.
Masking.

Missing
Full face smiles,
Laughing
Bodies

Jumping up and down,
Squealing,
Soulful Happy Huddle.

Infants deprived of
Human touch do not
Fare so well.

What about
Adults missing
Tender touch
Skin to skin?

Out of balance
With a natural
Love expression.

Cooties then.
Covid now.

We all became the little
Girls the boys didn't want
To touch.

LOVE AND LOSS

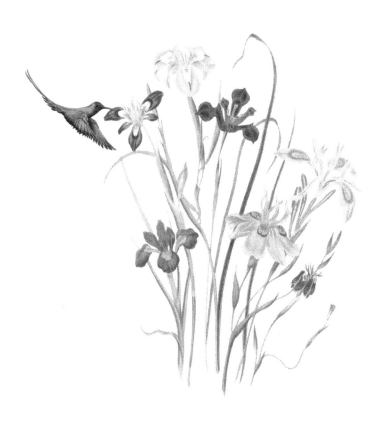

The Grieflove Place

May human beings find
Common ground
In the heartache
Of love
That death brings.
May streams of tears
Flow into the
Width of a
Roaring river,
Rocky cliffs, muddied banks,
Soft lily pads in a
Still lake of
Heart-centeredness,
With those we now see
Through
Wet eyes.

A world of trees,
Chilling harsh winds, drifts of snow,
Brilliant stars in a
Night sky.

Promises of bright, colorful
Flowers, bees,
Warm sunshine.

To weep, and
Meet one another in the
Grieflove place.

May heaving hearts
Reach an
Expansiveness,
A capacity to
Awaken
In unity,
Grace,
Humbled.
Inspired to
Live another
Sacred day of
Delicious life.

Wishes for You

May you know that Love remains the source of your life.

May you accept that there are no secret practices to protect you from heartbreak, that you simply must allow your heart to shatter into a zillion pieces over and over again to let all the gooey love in the center gush out into our world.

May you cultivate a deep, unwavering peace inside of you, unshakeable by all the noisy thoughts, external clatter, and cacophony of life.

May you be here now in this moment with no judgment, no expectations of Love showering you with money, things, or experiences with wonderful, self-aware people, with no gripping, clinging, grasping for what may not be meant for you or your soul's journey.

May you stay open to the experiences that are meant for you.

May you allow them to come in Love's time.

May you believe that those dreams deep inside of you continue to be heard even if you never create a collage, vision board, or declare it to the world. May you courageously clear away what needs to be released inside of you and outside of you because you know that these actions can completely transform your entire existence.

May you experience gratitude for all that is your life.

May you trust that love-fueled actions, creative expressions come from the silent places-the inhale of inspiration.

May you realize that you and your faith are writing the story of your life. May you realize that you will exit in the middle of the movie.

May you become a forever free being of love, kindness, tenderness, vulnerability, bravery, and compassion.

In My Bones

Almost lost you
Twice.
Your deep cries for
Help.
That aching
Loneliness
I heard
In my Bones.

Looking at you.
Buried in a blanket
On the floor.
You uttered lost
Hopeless words
Of desperation.

Your pain
Throws the
Ladder,
Clattering into the
Backyard.

Standing firm.
Dial numbers
Fingers for your life.

Seven Emergency
Vehicles,
Flashing Lights.
I count from
The flat roof
Strewn with crisp
Leaves on
Dark black rubber
Of that
Autumn day.

Burly Officers
Grab Hold
Either Side.
Your whole body
Swearing
Struggling.
Now unmoving,
Hunched in a red jacket
In the back seat
Of a police cruiser.
Stunned, barely breathing
In my bones.

In the wheelchair
Hospital gown,
Body
Void of Emotion,
Arm muscles
Showing.
Orderlies
Transport.
Mind fears I've
Lost you.
Heart says "no."

I Declare
Your
Thriving life.
Knowing
Unconditional
Mother love.
Unrelenting.
Unwavering.
Flowing fierce
In my bones.

Phones calls,
Meetings.
Remembering
You love

Wilderness.
Mountains
Winds, snow,
Tents, backpacks.
Wise people
Guide.

Honest
Raw
Real Letters
Pour out
Unedited.
Truth
Without blame
From you.

Then
Relocate to
A new life.
Relief mixed
With grief.

Missing you
Laughter, hugs,
Witty words
That smile
Not the empty
Alcoholic.

Star War
Legos,
Soft
Stuffed black
white cat,
An eagle with wings
Spread on
Your Dresser.
Reminders
Of a far away
Childhood,
Forever embedded
In my bones.

Phone rings.
Your
Vibrant voice
Sounds like
Love in my ears.
"I'm graduating
from high school!
I have a job,
benefits, 401K,
a car."
Weeping with joy
In my bones.

Hot sun,
Cool breeze.

A stadium full
Of strangers.
You in
Billowing bright
Cobalt blue,
Holding your cap
With golden tassel.
Cheering loudly.
Exuberance, pride,
Inspiration.
Private tears
In my bones.

That call
You shared
You helped a man.
He had no hands.
Bent over,
Eating the food
You had unwrapped.
Your voice cracked.
Choking on tears,
"I'm alive. I have hands.
I see I'm a spiritual
Being here to love and hold dear, a
Human
Experience.
What you've been telling me
All along is true."

You finally see what
I see has always been true,
As I celebrate you,
Your life
In the balance,
In my bones.

With Gratitude and Love for a Dog

A couple of years ago, my dog, Layla, walked across the rainbow bridge to be with her momma, Lynzeebear. I realized I've been fortunate to have dogs in my life for two decades. Our dogs Liesel, Socks, Lynzeebear, and Layla; woofed, wiggled and wagged in our life as a family. Layla remained a constant companion during the move from the family home to my Red Cardinal House, then to the House of Joy, as I created my new life in the mountains of North Carolina. By my side, Layla stayed as I grieved through losses and joys: including my son's abrupt departure to another state, Lynzeebear's death, my daughter's college years, her graduation, cherished friends' deaths, and the launch of three books. She walked with me during days and nights with the trees, bunnies, black bears on trails at Mount Mitchell and Craggy Gardens along the Blue Ridge Parkway.

Layla had arrived as a surprise gift for both of my children. They had been joking with me about my lack of spontaneity, which happened to be very accurate at that time. I remember thinking I'd show them how I could be spontaneous! Of course, a surprise involves implementing advanced logistics.

I picked up Layla during a dramatic thunderstorm of

falling branches, booming thunder, rapid flashes of lightning, pounding rain. I'm grateful both children were surprised. Yet, delight mixed with some disappointment when Layla showed her fears by barking incessantly at my daughter and then-husband. Once Layla realized that these two people loved her, that her pack had altered, she bonded beautifully with them.

A few weeks into our routines as a family with Lynzeebear and Layla, my daughter's junior year Prom Day arrived. In the late afternoon, her friends entered our home, the gathering location before photos. The door opened and closed many times on this gorgeous day in May. Guys in tuxedos, shiny shoes, girls with their hair, make-up, jewelry, flowing, colorful, beautiful dresses, high heels walked into the house along with parents wanting to take photos of their sons and daughters.

Lynzeebear began following me, but I didn't see Layla anywhere. I ran through the house looking for her, yelling her name. Layla was not in sight. My son and I ran out of the house calling "Layla!" while jogging up and down streets in our neighborhood. My heart pounded as I imagined the worst.

I returned to our house knowing that we needed to leave for the park to take photos. My daughter, her friends, and parents had gathered outside on the porch.

"Mom, didn't you find her?" my daughter asked.

I shook my head. Then I heard someone shout. "There she is!" I turned around. Proudly prancing up the driveway came Layla.

"Ugh. What is *that* in your mouth?"

The colorful, coiffed gathering of people screamed, squealed, and moved quickly inside the house. They closed the glass storm door behind them then turned around to stare at Layla. She carried a decomposing carcass of an animal. Was it a possum, a squirrel, a groundhog? Gross, putrid. Nasty. Foul-smelling. She dropped her prize at my feet, looked up. Her tail wagged and her eyes beamed. I scooped her up, opened the storm door as people made a wide path. I walked swiftly and placed her safely in her crate.

"I don't believe you'll ever be a hunter, Layla."

My then-husband begrudgingly removed the carcass from the porch. When that excitement passed, people walked to their vehicles to drive to the Park of Roses for photos. I climbed into the backseat with my daughter and son. My daughter's date rode shotgun. With relief, we talked and laughed hysterically about Layla's catch.

"Stop talking about that God Damn Dog!" My then-husband roared from the driver's seat.

We continued looking at each other with twinkling eyes, shoulders, and bodies shaking with suppressed laughter.

Dogs, pets of all kinds, teach us about patience and care in this interspecies dance of love. They become part of the rhythm and cycles of our lives. We do what seem like mundane routines of feeding, walking, scooping poop, petting, training, playing catch, bathing, and snuggling. Yet, woven into these tasks, we learn about simple acts of kindness. We notice the gentle nuance of their facial expressions, body movements, joy, and pain. Pets teach us a great deal about being humane, about unconditional love and loyalty. We bond with these sentient beings, forever a gift in our experience of being alive.

May you know the joy of having a pet or of loving animals of all kinds. May you know that the daily small tasks done with much care, tenderness, and mindfulness weave into a rhythm, a cycle of a life of unconditional love. May you experience the simplest moments linking together, creating a beautiful tapestry of a life worth living.

Story Interrupted

Divorce equals death.
A lie, a truth people
Tell themselves.
Justify walking away,
Turning their backs.
Tossing the Story of You
Like a notebook
Under a bus, rumbling
Down a muddy, dirt road.

Barriers go up to
Protect
Even though
Innocent children
Dance, play, weep
In backyards
Of two houses.

Adults hold tight to
Tribal righteousness

Family Loyalty
Disconnected from
Another
Human family.
Deluded into thinking
The Holy Grail of
Unconditional Love
Had been found.
A wishful, starry eyed hope
Projected onto imperfect beings.

Left behind
in
Desk drawers,
All your love notes,
Thank you
Cards,
Genuine gifts
From your heart.

Once an in-law,
Called an out-law,
Now
Cast out.

Pulling the half written
Manuscript off the
Muddy road, tire treads

Left behind on its back,
Marking the moment of
Departure.

Walking with this
Quiet ache of papers,
Yearning
For that human place of
Belonging in
A Hard Cover
Book.

Stained pages of the past
Catch the wind.

Each piece lifts off
Flies free in
Gusts
Carried
Far
Away.

Angels Lift All of You

You no longer
Lash out at me
With your viper
Tongue.
The spittle of
Jealous
Resentments
Escape
Late at night
In the early
Spring.
Your wounds,
My Inner critic.
My wounds,
Your inner bully.

Angels lift all of you.
An offering
From
A mushroom cloud of
Fury.

In the quiet of candles,
Burning on an altar,
Created as transition
Vigil.

Love songs now
Croon,
Swoon.
Holding soft petals,
With tiny dew droplets,
Like fresh seeds of nourishment.
Wafts of lavender relax
Gripping toes that
Held a lifetime of
Terror.
Touching
Fur on a dog's floppy ears.

Heaven sighs.

Wide open
In the midst
Of blooming crepe myrtle,
Bright yellow, petaled,
Black-eyed Susan,
Peeks at green peapods.

Honking geese splash
Landing in a lake.

A
Purified
Heart
Beats with
New Life.

The Might of Mercy

*I*n that miraculous way that only the universe can seem to create, I received mysterious mail with handwritten ink on the front, a small, note-sized envelope with the name I used during my second marriage. I opened it to discover that a woman is attempting to locate my first husband to unite him with some lost or unclaimed funds. I saw a number on the bottom of the sheet of paper. I chose to dial this number, which I will hang up if it feels like a scam. A woman answered.

"Hello, this is Laura Staley-my name is now Staley. You sent me a letter stating that you're attempting to locate my first husband."

"Yes. Let me get to my desk. Wait just a moment. (Pause) Here it is, yes. This is good news for him. He has an opportunity to claim funds that are legally his. Do you have his contact information? I have been attempting to notify him."

"He attended my father's celebration of life. My sister let me know because I had already left the event and missed interacting with him. I have his contact info, and I will reach out to him."

"That would be so helpful. Thank you. Kindly leave my number and name. Assure him that this is good news, that I'm legit."

"I will. Have a good day!"

I received a text that the two of them talked, that his mom, who I had loved, had recently died. I realized I still loved both my first ex and my former mother-in-law. I took a deep breath and tapped his number on my cell phone; we had not talked in years.

"Hello," he answered.

"Hello. This is Laura. I am so sorry to hear about the death of your mom. My heart is with you in your grieflove."

Thus began a sweeping share of his many recent health challenges and his doctor told him to get his affairs in order. He shared stories of his mother, ways he lovingly remembered me. Sprinkled through the conversation, I appreciated him; I let him know he was/is a good man. I shared that all those years ago, I had only scratched the surface of what became my deep, unrelenting work to heal, to transform.

I listened to his familiar voice from the depths of a quiet mind that I have cultivated over the years. With reverence and warmheartedness, a willingness I did not know I had, I heard him in a way I never could all those years ago. He shared that one of the best days of his life happened on the boat ride we took in Washington, D.C. I remembered the blue and white dress I wore, how I rushed to the bathroom immediately after he proposed and cried with mixed emotions. Some part of me screamed, "*Oh, God, No!*" while other parts of me, aching to be loved, said, "*Say, Yes!*" I knew he waited at the table for my return, for my answer. He had not gotten down on one knee. His proposal did not look like the movie script in my head. Many expectations roared at us from my parents, mostly my mother. I do not remember this day as one of the best of my life.

Hearing his voice through the phone, though his health was failing, I noticed his spirit remained strong, full of energy, expression, and humor. We laughed several times during our conversation. When we shared stories about his mother, we laughed and spoke our love then and now for her.

Oh, all these many deaths that keep happening. Arriving like constant ocean waves on the shore that don't ever cease, washing away the people we have loved, once loved, still love, will always love.

In the wake of ending an hour and a half time suspended like a long-held breath phone conversation, I sat quietly breathing. Tears streamed down my face. I felt forgiven, cherished. After I told him how his mother regularly told me how beautiful I was, even as I struggled to hear her, to let that kindness into my heart, he said,

"Please include me in the company of people who think you are beautiful."

Could I let his kind words seep through the last remnants of the protective wall I built around my unworthy of love young woman self, a self who got formed by too many unworthy younger selves? Will these parts of me ever cease to show up, cry out for genuine, kind love, sweet love?

Can I inhale and exhale love, mercy, kind compassion for a man at whom I screamed, "Fuck You!" all those years ago in a rage storm before squealing the tires of my vehicle as I drove away in pain and poisonous righteousness? During that time, I felt like a cornered animal terrified of love, thoroughly convinced of an impending loveless life. Had I not forgiven this earlier version of myself? This twenty something me felt so abandoned by love and too terrified to soften, yield, and receive. This younger version of myself had looked to him to meet the vast desert of thirsty, starving unmet needs, the love deprivation I had endured for far too long. No one man could ever have filled that bottomless well of need, of desire. *Forgive your younger wounded warrior who lived inside a battle for her heart, soul, mind, and freedom. Yes, I forgive younger me. He already has; maybe he did years ago.*

The might of mercy shows up once again to create deeper healing. He became the second person in a matter of weeks who appeared from the past who knew, saw, understood more than I realized at the time. In a box of memorabilia sent to me from my parent's house from my sister, I found a letter he wrote on my behalf to my mother. He never told me he had written this respectful request. He wrote asking that she find a way to love me, that he knew she could love me, that I deserved a mother's love. I realized he witnessed the words and deeds of my mother towards me. Fortunately, I got to thank him tearfully during our phone call for writing that letter so many years ago. He became another person who bore witness to the difficult reality I endured.

During this miraculous reconnection conversation with our brave and open hearts in a merciful place, I now can love him, soul untethered, till "death do us part."

You can shower people with love and kindness. If they haven't broken all the seashells of barrier reefs around their hearts and ground this into soft, porous sand, the love may not seep into the crevices and niches of the hurt, pain, their terror. The work must take place inside each person's soul as they gain a sense of safety inside their skin, uncoil, melt their protective shields, and heal their traumas. Over time, for some, in the space of many gentle showers of love, kindness, the soft underbelly of people may eventually appear, teary-eyed, receptive.

May you hear, express, and receive heartfelt realizations that might take years to see with open eyes and awakened whole hearts. May these expressions fill you to overflowing with compassion, tenderness and wet tears seeping into the soft sand footprints of lives transformed by grace.

Lungs for Life

Refusing to grieve is like avoiding
That belly expanding intake,
suppressing a huge sigh,
Fussing at the chaotic surface
Of shallow spasms.

Grieving is deep breathing.
Body breathing is living.
Living means loving, losing, releasing
What was not ever yours to keep in
Those clenched hands, pursed lips,
Steeled heart.

Expand your torso.
Open your heart.
Breathe, flutter, grieve.

Inhale and be.
Exhale and cry.
Inhale and love.
Exhale and live.

Rest. Move. Play.
Create.

Live this
Day in Love.
One
Aware breath
Deepening into
The next awakened
Conscious breath of your
Beautiful, most wondrous,
Miraculous Life.

Remembering Maribeth

*W*hile running by the river a few years ago in the midst of my life turning inside out and upside down, I noticed another woman runner. She looked familiar to me, and as she ran closer, I recognized and remembered who she was. She recognized me, too. We stopped and began excitedly talking at the same time.

"It's so great to see you! Oh my gosh, how are you?!?!"

She admitted that this was the first time she'd ever run in this neighborhood. She liked running outside but usually drove to a fitness center to work out. I shared that I ran almost every single day on this path.

We had met several years ago when she facilitated seminars for transformational trainings in which I had participated. I felt the warm rush of gratitude all over again for her guidance, wisdom, and coaching. Her bright yellow running jacket complimented her smile, presence, beauty, and radiant energy on that dark, cloudy, cold, early spring day.

She asked about my life. I told her my marriage had ended, that I was selling the house and moving to another house in this same neighborhood. Hearing about my divorce, she noted that her long-term relationship had also come to an end. Since her break-up, she had met another love.

"When are you moving, Laura? I can help you move!"

"At the beginning of May, and that would be great. I'd love your support. That's kind of you to offer! Thank you, Maribeth!"

We exchanged contact information along with a hug and more words of what a wonderful surprise to see each other again.

Moving day arrived. The sun shone brightly through clear blue skies that morning. She drove up and got out of her compact car. We hugged each other. I introduced her to my friends, my daughter, who had just completed her freshman year in college, and her friends. I felt this overwhelming sensation of love for all these wonderful people who had generously shown up to help me alongside my focused "Let's Move!" self. Much squealing and hugging took place as we gathered ourselves together.

When the young men from Two Men and a Truck pulled up, the moving party began. I felt the excitement in the air as all these young people-the movers and my daughter and her friends seemed to notice one another in a kind, celebratory way. Some innocent flirting likely took place.

Friends commented on how incredibly organized I was. Stacked labeled boxes filled the living room, ready for departure. The grab, load, and go began in earnest. The movers loaded the large furniture and containers onto the truck. The rest of us loaded vehicles and a pick-up truck. Everyone knew their tasks.

By noon, my kitchen had been unpacked by my daughter and her friends. At this juncture, I offered all my team food. Maribeth declined. Instead, she made another generous offer.

"I would like to mow your front yard."

Like every person in the entire neighborhood, she had noticed the knee-high grass mixed with thousands of dandelions in both the large front yard and the bowling alley back yard. Renters had vacated the house in November. The previous owner lived out of state and had hired people to do only the bare minimum to sell the house.

"Really?" I didn't have much experience with this chore. My son and his dad had been the lawnmowers at the family house.

"Hey, Laura, I *love* to mow lawns! I mow the lawn at my house. I really would like to do this for you, but I need to change into other clothes because it's gotten really hot."

"Okay. Thank you so much, Maribeth! Again, this is such a kindness. I appreciate this. I will get the lawnmower out of the garage for you."

Those who could stay ate pizza and drank water or soda on the back patio.

Maribeth returned and mowed the front yard until the electric mower's battery needed recharging. I thanked her, hugged her, and promised to take her to lunch with the other friends who hadn't been able to stay for pizza.

Four of us, including Maribeth, met a couple of months later for lunch, laughed a great deal about the move, and updated one another on good things in our lives. Happy to treat these dear friends to a meal, I felt much joy and gratitude for the ways they had shown up for me.

Maribeth and I promised to stay in touch after that lunch. A few months flew by. On a cold February morning close to Valentine's Day, I received a call from a cherished long-time friend, who had helped me on moving day and laughed with me during that lunch gathering.

"Laura, you probably want to sit down. I have awful news. Maribeth is dead. She was murdered. I know you don't watch the news and probably don't want to. I just knew I needed to call you as soon as I heard. She was stabbed to death in her own home. There were no signs of breaking and entering. She likely knew the suspect. The story is all over the local news stations and on Facebook. I knew you'd want to know. I'm so sorry. This is so unbelievably tragic."

I could barely breathe. The shock left me almost speechless. Finally, some words spilled out of me.

"I'm so grateful you called. Thank you for being the person I am hearing this news from. Oh, I'm stunned. I love you so very much. I love you so very much. Oh, kind, loving Maribeth. Oh. Oh. Oh. Thank you for calling. I love you."

"I love you so much, too, Laura. We'll talk real soon. I will see you at the library on Thursday morning."

I had no idea Maribeth lived at risk of death, let alone murder. I knew so little. She is the only person I know who has died so violently. The difficult process of accepting her death continues even after a handful of years have passed. By sharing I celebrate her life, her love, her kindness, the earth angel she was, and now the heavenly angel she will always be. By choosing to be kind to other people and remembering the many positive ways she touched my life and many other people's lives, I honor Maribeth. I will always remember her.

May you know how precious life really is. May you graciously receive the kindness of friends and give generously of your talents while you are here. May you break your silence if you suspect domestic violence.

Fallen and Risen

I have fallen and risen, fallen and risen, fallen and risen a million times; to discover that I have fallen and risen in love with the experience of being alive. No matter the size of the ocean waves, the rolling tides of uncertainty, the crashing thunderstorms, lightning strikes, and doubtful all-day sunshiny, blue skies filled with hope. The ducklings arrive and hide underneath their mama duck for safety, then venture out for a meal of tiny bugs, to groom their downy, fuzzy bodies, huddle together, and learn to glide through calm waters.

Can you trust the goodness of life, your ever-evolving body of wisdom, your ability to adapt, pivot, reframe, shift, adjust, swim, and create? You are still *here*. You must've figured some stuff out.

Unblocking the Heart as Life Flows

My adult daughter's birthday this year became the first in which we were not together. Anticipating this, I called her.

Grasping for ideas, forgetting I was talking to a twenty-something, I blurted,

"Maybe we could do a Zoom Bananagrams game or Zoom dancing together! I just don't want a five-minute phone call. I know you have a full adult life. I honor that, but I want to celebrate you! I'm your mom!"

"Mom, during the week, I'll likely have dinner with my dad, then a lunch with my aunt, and drinks and a meal with my friends. I'm disappointed we will not be together, but I understand. Mostly, I look forward to when we can be with each other."

"I do too. I love you."

"I love you so much, mom."

Then a fabulous idea downloaded. *I can create short videos in which I share stories and memories of my daughter each day for a week and send these to her!* I joyously began this process.

Two days before my daughter's special day, Layla, the dog I had gifted both of my children seven years ago, died.

Determined to stay in the joy amidst my sorrow, I

continued recording whatever bubbled up. I included thoughts about her essential character qualities, her delightful, sassy personality, things she had said-all woven in a stream of tears, smiles, laughter-a treasure trove of memories that remain on an internal love-filled DVR.

On the evening of her birthday, I received an unexpected phone call.

"Mom! I had an amazing birthday!"

Her exuberance burst my heart wide open. She excitedly shared the ways she had been loved, cherished, celebrated. She adored the videos.

"Oh, I love you so much, Momma!"

"Happy Birthday, Sweetheart! I love you forever and always!"

In the days that followed her birthday, waves of grief arrived at all the expected and unexpected moments. In the absence of Layla, the silence felt deafening.

I noticed stragglers-like hidden, lonely, crinkled letters, yellowed photos, and sparkling silver charms from a bracelet, climbed on board a precarious, slippery surfboard of my sorrow. I rode the waves of loss with memories of both my parents, who died during this last year, of not knowing when I would get to be with both my adult children, the three of us together. Unresolved grief persisted in piggybacking like thick blankets layered on top of an already heaving heart.

Edgy agitation began to build in my body. I couldn't sit still to get any given task done from beginning to end-even simple ones. I wanted to jump outside of myself with all this loss.

While pedaling my bicycle the next day on a crisp autumn morning, I remembered a friend's essay about finding her joy in drawing, collaging, and another friend who drew stick figures to process her emotional realities.

That evening I clicked on music I love, pulled out white sheets of paper, markers, and colored pencils. I cried, created, and colored a drawing; unremarkable, yet filled with different parts of me. The process opened me in places I didn't even realize were blocked. I remembered that life is messy, full of celebrations and loss and the importance of feeling everything, taking out all the thorns to heal. While drawing, I discovered a comforting place for my younger selves to mourn and celebrate, for my adult self to be uninhibited, free.

I noticed when several beloved ones die within a short time frame amid life's joyous occasions, you can either: distract yourself by binge drinking, eating, shopping, stuffing the feelings in boxes that you carry to a dark basement, or by courageously feeling the layers and depth of loss. You can engage beneficial modalities for releasing sorrow, love, and joy.

Many of you are filled with emotional pain, which you can no longer numb, avoid, or suppress because you have awakened to the fact that you want to live, that your soul deserves a chance to breathe, to dance.

How important to find ways to feel... All of It. How meaningful to hear a sage voice inside say,

"Welcome to living life as a human being who feels, who experiences what it means to be alive, who embodies radical empathy and exudes love."

What will be born from our sorrows, our joys, our loves, from the brave releasing of a life we no longer live?

Being present moment by moment as best you can for what can seem like a deluge of heart-wrenching experiences mixed with joyous, simple ones of celebration, life continues to flow. Hospice and midwifery happen simultaneously inside and outside of us.

Keeping your heart open means allowing life to flow through-to leave tiny love notes, soft, tender touches, drawings as a trail that leads us to appreciate the tears of a thousand losses. Those sorrows often become seeds that grow loving-kindness trees in the center of our vast, ever-expanding, beautiful souls.

May we remain connected in our mourning, in our joyful celebrations, and in the metamorphosis of who we are becoming individually and collectively. May as many of us as possible become alchemists for love.

A Visit

Sitting
In
The seat
Of the soul.
Quiet
Witness.
Voyeur of
Body Sensations.
Gurgling
Intestines.
Abdomen
Expanding.
Relaxed
Mouth
Tongue
Wet
Eyes soft.
Clothing closely
Nestling skin.

Sunshine
Streams through a
Window.

Your Voice
Echoes
Warm internal
Shower.
Tingles
Like
An
Electric
Current.
Ah…
Your
Love
Visiting from
Beyond.

Acceptance

The wild geese
Honk in rhythmic beat.
Wings pulsing on the wind.
A feathered V formation.
Velveteen black
Stretched necks
Soar.

Red cardinals with
Their lovely mates
Cheer, cheer, cheer
Beside a
Window.
A reminder
To sing a song
Every single day.

Butterflies land
On hands,
Shoulders,
Crown Chakra,

Purple cornflowers.
Soft, fragile,
Enduring,
Beautiful symbols of
the capacity to
Transform.

Babies
Laugh, giggle,
Chortle
Cry, weep,
Wail
Slobber
Drool.
Watch through
Eyes filled with
Wonder.

Lovers
Passionately kiss
Like the First kiss,
The last kiss.

Beloved ones
Hold one another
In joy,
In celebration.

Sunshine
Streams through
Windows,
Reflects
Rippling, dancing sparklers
Flashing diamonds,
A light show
On the lake.

People
Laugh. Infectious,
Caught in quick
Bursts of
Breath.

Eating, sleeping,
Lovemaking,
Cooking.
Gathering
Ingredients.
Sipping coffee,
Tea.

Bustling
Bravely on.
People
Go about
Their days,
Nights.

Here I sit.
Not ever again
Able to tell
You,
"I love you."
No last chance
To feel your
Always warm
Hand holding
Mine.

Your gentle
Voice
Speaks
Inside the
Place where
I wove you
Round and round
My heart.

ABUNDANT HEART

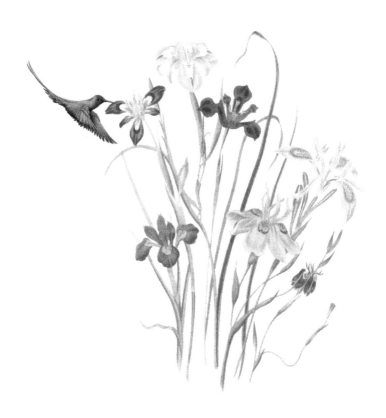

Heartwarming Calls

I called my poet friend to let her know what I loved about the poem she had written. She sent it through our group email because we had to maintain a safe distance during this unprecedented time of Covid19. Her soft, sweet voice burst with joy as she shared about the lunch-warm chicken and food from The Bistro; she had eaten outside on a glorious, warm spring day.

"Oh, Laura, the trees are so *beautiful*-all the flowering blossoms in pinks and whites-the gorgeous yellow of the forsythia!"

Her joyful energy flowed around me, lifting me. I shared how much I love the blue sky, white clouds, and those delightful pops of color emerging after the more monochromatic winter hues.

I let her know that my mom had died two days ago. I told her I had cried a bit when I realized I would never hear my mother say these words: "I'm proud of you. I accept you exactly as you are." Alive, she had not been able to utter those phrases. My friend knew the challenging, complicated relationship I had navigated with my mother.

"Laura, your mom is proud of you. She loves you

completely now. She *is love!* Her spirit is *love.* Love is all there is!"

Tears welled up in my eyes as I realized the truth of the words spoken with hearty enthusiasm, faithful certainty from this wonderfully wise, cherished friend. We talked a bit more about the beautiful day outside, the rebirth of spring.

In my mind's eye and my sensed experience, I can remember her warm arms around me, the wisps of her long white hair as they lightly touch my face. I can see her bright eyes behind her glasses, her soft wrinkles around her glowing smile. We end the conversation with several "I love you's." and "I will talk to you soon!" flowing in and out like the tai chi movement Wave Hands Like Clouds.

I thought I would be the one to brighten my friend's day. Instead, I experienced an energy current of pure positivity from her precious soul whooshing through the phone and landing directly in my heart and body. It reminded me of the glowing alien in the movie "Cocoon" who sends loving energy to the human male character across the swimming pool, brightening his whole body with white expanding light.

Calling to hear a beautiful voice, the smile that enlivens the vocal cords, the lilting, tinkling, or booming chest resonance of human laughter can be essential emotional nourishment. Hearing the tone, cadence of the voice of a friend, colleague, neighbor, or beloved one energizes the entire heart, mind, body, and spirit. The content of the conversation doesn't even matter as the words ebb, flow, wiggle, trickle around each other in between the breaths of air inhaled, exhaled, exchanged back and forth like a delicious syllable waltz to the silent music of compassionate, caring presence.

May you take a moment to reach out with a heartwarming call to another human being or as many people as you choose. May this experience awaken you and power up your life force energy with love and joy reminding you that you matter, that human connections matter immensely and always have. May this become a delightful practice for as many days that you are blessed with precious life.

Delightful Surprise

Frozen
Wispy
Feather wings
On my
Blessed Blue's
Windshield.

White
Tiny
Leaf
Rubbings.

A
Snow fairy
Child's
Overnight
Art project.

December Chicks

Mama Duck
Stands out,
White with
Mottled brown
Feathers,
Bright orange
Legs.
Her four chicks
Peep, peep, peep,
Paddling
Behind her.

A colorful tapestry
Of bright yellow,
White, black.
Riding
Ripples of
Water,
Crafted
By the
Blustery

Late autumn
Wind.

A family
Together for a
Cell phone
Photo click,
Wisp of a
Moment.

A red-tailed
Hawk
Sits on
A grey thick branch
Up in a naked
Tree.

Mama Duck
And the
Hawk
Made
Arrangements
Long ago.

How
Fleeting the
Moments
Of being
A family.

How important to
Savor
Those
Snapshots.

New Parent

Welcome, precious one!
I love you
With
All that I am.

Curious to
Discover
Who You
Are.

What do
You love?
Are there thoughts
Inside your
Sweet, tiny head?
What makes
You
Smile,
Laugh,
Sigh, coo?

You wail and writhe.
Day and night.
Hot tears
Stream down
Both our cheeks.
Holding you.
Carrying you
Close heart to
Heart.

Singing
Songs
With words,
LaLaLa's
Calm
Both of us.
Hips swaying
A figure eight.
Gentle bounce,
Mom groove.

Drinking you
In.
Wide Eyes.
Nuzzling,
Tenderly
Touching
Your soft skin.

Feeling your
Tiny warm fingers
Grasp ahold of
My pinkie
Finger.

Nourishing your
Heart, mind,
Body, Soul.
Now settling down
For a much
Needed nap in
Love's Soft
Lap.

Spirit Animals

Each of you
Appears at just
The right moment.

Hummingbird
Whirring wings
Distinct from the
Buzzing bees.

A fleeting, enduring reminder.
Love life.
Sip nectar.
Move towards
Goodness.

Black Bears
Hibernate.
Look inside
A Den of your
Heart for Honey

Wisdom that's
Sticky Sweet.

Red cardinals
Show up brightly,
Bravely with your
Beautiful song.
Sing.

Painted Turtle.
Move slowly,
Patiently.
Pause in the tall
Grass. Breathe
Deeply inside
A Safe Thick
Decorative
Shield.

Sleek Doe
With large,
Brown eyes.
Never underestimate
Tenderness,
Gentleness,
Sensitivity.

Joy bursts
Wide open,

Reclaiming a
Little girl's
Delight
At the sight
Of all of you.

A
Woman
Blossoms,
Nurtured
Inside her
Natural
Habitat.

Synchronicities

During the dark days of winter, while navigating my divorce and worrying about my teen son, I saw a red cardinal outside the kitchen window. "Hello, Helen," I heard myself say out loud.

Red cardinals reminded me of the sweet elderly neighbor who lived next to us when my children were young. Helen loved cardinals. She filled almost every surface of her home with red cardinals of all shapes, sizes, and material, including cardinal sun catchers in every window. She often spoke of her passion for this gorgeous bird. Soon after we moved to a new house nearby, Helen died.

I knew I'd be selling the current family home in the spring. I thought briefly about the house where we lived next to Helen and how much I enjoyed our former neighbors, a community of good, caring people.

Months later as the daffodils bloomed and trees budded, I ran by our former house and noticed a "For Sale" sign in the yard of what used to be Helen's home. My realtor's company name was on the sign. Chills ran through my body.

Could this be my new home?

Doubt and fear quickly followed.

I have never owned a home by myself; I probably cannot afford it.

I dismissed the idea.

The family house sold in four days. I now had 30 days to locate a new place for my son and me to live.

"Mom, I do **not** want to live in a different community. I love this area and want to be close to my friends," my son cued me with his strong preference.

In my mind, images of the street where we used to live kept appearing. I wondered, again, about where we would live. I spoke with my realtor.

"I need a home to rent or possibly purchase. My son and I want to stay in the area. "

"Well, there's this house that we thought would sell quickly, but it has not sold, and I thought you might want to take a look at this property because you could afford to buy it and not have to rent."

I interrupted him. A warm tingling danced throughout my body.

"I know the house you are speaking of. It didn't sell because it's supposed to be mine."

He confirmed the address. He was describing the red cardinal house.

I met my realtor on a grey, rainy day during my son's spring break. I immediately fell in love with all the wood, the natural light through the many windows. How inviting it felt on such a dark day! My son walked through the house the next evening and loved it, too, especially the large backyard. He saw all kinds of possibilities.

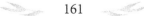

An offer remained on the table that came in lower than the asking price. My realtor and I wrote up an offer of $100.00 over. Not sleeping later that night, I picked up my phone and noticed a text from my realtor.

"Honey, congratulations, you're in contract!"

Overjoyed, I met the banker and filled out lots of paperwork. The banker, kind, transparent, and trustworthy, thoroughly explained everything. I listened intently and competently tracked everything he said. No longer seeing myself through other people's narrow and unkind perceptions, I smiled brightly. Filled with gratitude for my dad, I let everyone know at the closing about what my dad had meant to me as the person who taught me to live within my means, to pay bills in full. Having heeded my dad's financial wisdom, I had created the opportunity to be a homeowner as a single woman.

I celebrated this milestone with a delicious meal at one of my favorite healthy food restaurants, and then I returned to a street and community of neighbors I always loved.

Two of my best friends arrived as the first guests at Red Cardinal House. One gifted me a flag of a red cardinal, which I hung on the front door as a greeting. The other brought jewelry she made as gifts. Our celebration turned into a coming-out party as I modeled outfits my daughter had enthusiastically selected and encouraged me to purchase. My daughter had been eager to outfit me since she was in middle school. The excessive turtlenecks and zip-up hoodies plopped into donation bags as I began building a professional and casual wardrobe filled with feminine yet professional outfits.

My best friends assured me that I looked beautiful in these outfits and the dangling, new earrings. I laughed and wept. I felt beautiful for the first time in my adult life from the inside out. The transformation of every single aspect of my life continued.

My new home needed tender, love, and care after a series of renters had lived there. I took action every day removing most of the previous residents' belongings from the basement and garage. I hired contractors to build a fence, paint the walls, repair plumbing fixtures and pipes, and install a light and fan appliance over the stove. My empowered focus included actions for Cherish Your World, my professional company, and the growth of my "inner fly on the wall," that witness consciousness, what some call their Inner Knowing or Tabitha. Inspired, I played music I love. I kept writing. I savored cooking and eating healthy food. I continued running, dancing, grieving, and growing.

During a powerful, brave dance of deep transformation, an inner beauty burst out of me. Almost every aspect of my life shifted while the woman who looked back at me from the mirror evolved.

Like the gorgeous red cardinals that attract people's eyes and attention, I excitedly walked into the world to inspire others generously, gently, and lovingly on their journeys of transformation. These traits humbly remain my deepest purpose and passion, the legacy I want to leave.

If you happen to be walking through dark nights or months of your soul, I encourage you to gently broaden your perspective. Pay attention to tiny signs and synchronicities that can open doors to new possibilities. The natural world, especially, remains filled with flora and fauna that might point the way to your deepest heart's desires or remind you of the wisdom a beloved one shared with you.

My friend and colleague, Carol, describes these beautiful clues as divine breadcrumbs that you can trust and follow. Another colleague, Melissa, shares that luck can be cultivated, with optimism for the future, gratitude for what you do have, open-mindedness about opportunities, and an enjoyment of meeting new people.

My beloved friend Ruby calls this "divine choreography."

A beautiful dance can take place among inner dreams, kind people, tiny, beautiful signs, and brave, heartfelt actions to create astonishing transformations in real-time and actual places. Love always finds a pathway home.

May you see beautiful signs all around you. May you bravely take those heart and gut cued actions even when your mind might blather doubt and disbelief. May light from the sun meet you every day to remind you that sunshine touches everyone and everything, including you.

Compassionate Champion

No matter how
Many times
You get knocked down,
You rise strong.
Unrelenting,
Persevering,
Fierce in the face
Of dishonesty,
Dysfunctions.

Committed to integrity,
Transformations for
The quality of
People's lives-babies, children, adults.
You bring keen intellect,
Wisdom, life experiences,
Diligent research, and training to
Complex challenges and
Create
Processes that resolve issues

A meaningful
Invention.

Energy worker,
Beloved Friend,
Home Girl.
Experiencing respite,
Safe space
Compassion,
Grace in
Your presence.

A fiery, intentional
Commitment
To a joy
In being alive.
No matter what
Has come before
Us or
What comes
After us.
Seeing the
Strength
Resilience
Feeling resonance.

Whole Real
Hugs,
Belly laughter

Bonfires,
Bonding.
A Thanksgiving
With you,
Your family,
Embracing
Belonging
Believing.

Walking with
Roses.
Creating beauty
With jewels.
Loving your
Children and grands.
You are a champion,
Expanding a Legacy
Of Love, spirit,
Healing.

Beautiful, Gentle Friend

Standing next to
You on a playground
Feels so fine.
Our daughters
Bond in friendship,
Our lives intertwine.

Our families intersect
Through
Summers at
Our swimming pool,
Potlucks,
School Events.

Our children
Play together.
Imagination
Laughter
Creativity
Joyful expression,

Adventures and
Blanket tents.

Holidays bring
Us together.
Fourth of July.
Halloween.
Christmastime.
Beautiful memories
We create in
Clintonville.

Our mom friendship
Deepens through
Dark days of
Loss and grieving.
Sunny days of
Celebrations,
Milestones
Transitions
Fresh beginnings still.

Maggie, Liesel,
Lynzee, and Socks
All romp on the
Other side.
Jessie, Stewie,
Layla wag and

Woof. Cody struts.
A passion for
Pets we share.

Our children
Mature,
Pursue different
Paths,
We continue to care.

We remain close
As my life implodes.
Your unwavering presence,
Compassion creates
Safe space for
Anger, fears, tears.
Courage knowing
I could call you.
I do, many times.

Not alone on
Christmas Day.
Greeted with hugs.
You and your
Family's kindness
Wraps me in a
Present of love,
Sweet and sublime.

I see
Your ways of
Caring,
Embracing others
With openness
Grace.
Joy running
Obstacle courses
With pups.
Celebrating my new
Significant one.

Now residing in
Different states.
Me on a mountain.
You in a gorgeous
Ravine, delighting in
Your growing grandson.

The gift of our
Friendship endures.
In my mind's
Eye, I see
Your beautiful self,
Though we are apart.
I hear your
Laugh,
Imagine your quiet

Being.
Everyday grateful for you,
My beautiful, gentle
Friend.
Always in my heart.

Autumn Rose

Surrounded by
Colorful leaves
Fluttering away
From their stable
Tree branch homes.
A brief liberation
Before lying down,
Layered crimson, burnt red, golden
Blankets on the
Ground beneath.

You,
Bloom
Above.
Pink Beauty
Awakened,
Humbled
By Rain.

Are you
Whispering a tender

Prayer for
Humanity?

Remember,
Life still bursts
Forth during
Shorter days,
Longer dark nights
Of the Soul.

Then even
You,
Sweet
Darling,
Drop
Soft, dewy
Fragile petals,
With quiet
Dignity.
Knowing
That exquisite
Moment of
Graceful
Surrender
Into
Wintertime
Incubation.

Will we not
Trust the
Cycles of
Budding, blooming,
Bowing, and shedding
In our thousand
Times a thousand
Fresh day beginnings,
Endings?

Teach us,
Gentle
Autumn Rose.

The Peacemaker

Your gentle way of being
In the world,
I noticed the first time
We met at a juncture not
Knowing our fates.

I discovered you'd be
Someone I'd
Bring a
Casserole to
If something happened
To our respective
Mates.

Then it
Did.
Our friendship
Strengthened
As we found
Sea legs amidst
All the tides

Of change,
In a sea filled
With unfamiliar fish.

A cuddle buddy
You became.
Bonding in the kitchen
As sous chef
And chef
Of delicious
Vegan food.
Watching football,
Movies.
Brought chocolate
Instead of the covered dish.

Appreciating
Your space of
Dining.
Sacred shrine.
Comfy couch.
Cozy
Handholding,
Warm hugs.

Meaningful
Conversations
About Love,
Dating,

Life aspirations,
And loved ones
Addictions to drugs.

Inspiring me
To mediate,
To open my heart to
The impermanence of life.
To grow beyond
Aversions and attachments.
To be the observer,
The listener to the messages
From life.

We showed up
For each other
In ways that healed
And transformed.
In your eyes I
Found complete
Acceptance,
Unconditional Love,
A presence that pours
Into the soul
Of creativity,
Beauty and strife.

Walking humbly,
Quietly,

With a passion.
You are
A Bodhisattva
For loving-kindness.
A maker of peace.
An artist with
Enduring Compassion.

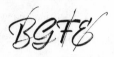

BGFE

You utter these first words
As you
Prep and paint,
"I have a big heart."
As though this was a flaw,
But it's your
Very essence.

You listen with
Presence as I
Pour out my rage,
Wreckage,
Resilience from
An Implode of life
As I knew it.

"There is little
That offends me."
This truth of how you
Live and care

For others
Frees me.

You answer
Curious questions
With an easy
Openness that surprises.
Not mincing words,
Or tiptoeing around
Difficult experiences.

We find respite in
Discovering similar
Values, interests,
Wounded places with
Compassion.

You become my muse,
A haven and playground
For an imagination
To come alive.
A poet begins to
Emerge.
With you,
I feel youthful,
Alive,
Hilarious,
Unleashed.

Transcending
What seemed like
Attraction,
We discover a
World of
Acceptance,
Heart-centered support,
Unrelenting encouragement,
Laughter.
Tears and cheers
For more of life's BS,
Accidents,
Stepping up,
Stepping out.

We share
Books, insights,
Revelations,
Wonderings and WTFs?!

Our ways of being
With each other
Build a bridge
To an enduring respect,
A multi-faceted love.

Forever grateful
For this forgiving friendship,
That allows us to be

Fully ourselves.

Seen.

Recognized.

Celebrated.

Together we create

A place where a passion

For ideas, a joy in being alive,

Honesty, vulnerability

Expands

In this

Crazy, beautiful life.

Belong to the Creek

Struggling into bright colored tights.
Itchy, scratchy crinolines.
Stiff, shiny, slippery bottomed shoes.
Suffocating adult expectations.
Nice clothes could not
Get muddy, torn, soaked.

Defiant, shrieking, laughing
Stomping in mud puddles.
Running towards the
Babbling brook.
Attempting a crawdad catch.
Delighting in skating bugs
Visible on a
Sunlit, sparkling, conveyor belt.

Play clothes drenched.
Sitting cross-cross applesauce
on smooth flat underwater
Stones.
Hands and arms hover

Still
Above the liquid swirls.
Moss-covered faces
smile at this sublime
partial submersion.

Milky blue sky,
boulders, the small turtle
Climbing slowly on top of a rock that
Stands dry above the gurgling,
Retracts its snake-like head inside skin layers,
An artfully designed, yellow and black shell.
Slowly its
Eyes seek
To look,
Safe to wonder what
Captivates
A sun, water drenched
Beaming, bright-eyed girl.

Spider Webs

Fragile, sturdy, delicate strands
Thinner than dental floss,
Astonish.
Seemingly invulnerable to rain or wind,
These creations-
The ones right outside the door
Remain utterly untouched.
Intricate in their mandala weave-like way.
Waiting,
Gentle nets to capture nourishment.
Works of art by tiny creatures
Whose lives can quickly be extinguished
By unaware human beings
Caught in mental tangles of angst.

Can we pause?
Pay rapt attention?

What are we creating
That's tender, resilient

Precious, life-giving,
Impermanent to
Our own existence?

Glistening Diamond

We meet each other
Years ago, at
Coffee shops,
Mexican restaurants.
Accurate rumors of
Your magnificence
Proceed before
I formally greet you.

Discovering similar
Childhood into
Adulthood training in
Superpowers of
Deflecting projections,
extracting
Introjections,
We bond in
The goo.

Holding each other
To our highest and best
Becomes our clear
Commitment.
Knowing many
Transformations
Will manifest and
They do.

Brilliant storyteller.
Dissector of people,
Dynamics using
Ketchup bottles,
Saltshakers,
Sugar packets.
Sniffing out the
Deeper patterns
Undercover,
Seemingly stuck like
Glue.

Listening for
Commitments
Others hold
In their hearts.
Wise to the
Wider context,

Impacts,
Implications,
Your keen
Intuition
Sings.

Halloween,
Your favorite
Holiday.
Elaborate costumes,
Lively parties,
Now a double
Treat Birthday
For cake and
Spooky bling.

Powerfully dynamic,
Colorful
Vivacious
Hilarious
Gorgeous.
Shining bright
Like a
Glistening Diamond.
Enduring
With love
My best friend
Forever
Flourishing.

Loving Soul Twin

Instant
Connection
Like I've known
You for a lifetime.
We quickly discover
Common history,
Childhoods,
Adulthoods,
Common themes,
Courageous daring.

Our sons'
Topsy turvy
Paths.
Brilliant minds,
Shining Hearts,
Bodhisattvas.
Our daughters
Fierce for Integrity,
Truth and caring.

We co-create
Lovely lyrics
Someday may
Be sung.
A Template
For transformations.
A story board,
Such ease.

Traveling to
NYC,
Earth angels
Gather.
Open-hearted,
Going with the flow.
Meditating
Connecting
Laughing.
United Nations
International
Day of Peace.

Standing in sunshine,
Rain, snow,
Wind, cold.
Wearing
boots,
Scarves, gloves

At the intersection
For love,
Such a breeze.

Seeing, speaking
Feeling
Relishing
Riffing
Crying
Holding
Each other
Close
Cups
Of hot tea.

Sparkling
Fairy Hair
Lively
Vibrant.
Freely
Walking with
Elves.

Kindness,
Compassion in your
Magic wand.
Bristling demeanors soften
In your presence.

A generous guide to
Our healthiest,
most creative
Selves.

Unwavering instrument,
A channel,
Caring for others.
You sow
Scrumptious seeds
Thought, word
And deed.

Embodied
Love in
Action.
Beautiful heart.
Gorgeous soul.
Infectious laugh,
Warm hugs,
A welcome home
Whenever.

Bursting with joy,
I knew
Loving
Soul twin,
Beloved One

Cherished friend.
A rich gift,
A treasure
Forever.

Rushing Waters

Rushing waters towards deeper places.
Rolling into low ground,
Seeping into soil.
Liquid freedom moving, flowing, roaring.
You can hear the pitter, patter
From enclosed spaces.

Are you drowning in the rainy days?

Earth gets a drink,
Now intoxicated.

Many pints poured down the throat,
From a grey furrow of shadowy foreheads.
Brows turned towards each other
In angst and anguish.

Wishing for an umbrella sky of hope.

Passionate cloud kisses
Filled with love flowers.

Silent Snow

Soft
Upper Palette.
Juicy Tongue
Touches
Relaxed Lips.
Skin supple,
A soft
Blanket over
Muscle and bone.
Sinking,
Melting
All the way
To the warm
Chair.

Aware
Right here.
Hearing
Furnace blower
Whir.

Snow falling
Softly on the ground,
Outside these large
Windows.
Powdered sugar
From a Sky White
Distant
Heavenly Grandma,
Adding the last
Touches on her
Frozen earth cake.

Cooler air entering
Nostrils.
Warmer air
Exiting.

Was going
To go
Grocery shopping.

Rather sit
Here
Holding
A quiet mind
Breathing
With silent
Snow.

Sparkling Earth Angel

It feels like you've
Been part
Of me and in
My heart for a
Lifetime.

Grateful for
Your deep listening,
Ability to
Hold space for
Tears, fears, anger,
Jubilation.
Evolutions in
The midst of
Change and springtime.

Inviting many
To dance, meditate,
Celebrate.
To evolve through

Stages of healing
In our bones,
Muscles, breath,
And with art.

Creating a group,
A gathering for support,
For love, compassion,
Non-judgment,
Our highest and
Best. Inspired Souls
Rise strong because of
Your commitment and
Passion to hold the heart.

You see beyond
Profanity, the past,
And imperfections.
You show up for life,
Friends, family, my
Beloved ones and me in
Meaningful ways that
Take me to my knees with
Heartfelt appreciation.
With you I find
Safe space to be celebrated,
Uplifted, and loved no matter
What curve balls come.

With you in my life
I experience less
Trepidation.

Beauty,
Grace, Care,
Kindness,
A goddess
Attracting
Stars, flashes,
Sun beams, and
Strength.

You are a
Gift, a treasure,
A Connector for those who
Feel lost, coming apart,
Or all alone without a
Home. This lives powerfully
In your everyday actions
Effortlessly
Tending to others at length.

Your lilting laughter,
Smiling face,
Flowing hair,
Graceful being
Dancing with wings,

Running with clarity,
Soaring with love, inspiration,
Delight.
You, Earth Angel,
Bless us all with
The wonder of your
Sparkling light.

Oh, This Love

Singles mingle
A Westerville
Bar and Grill.
I swear you
Twinkled at
Me.
You emailed me
For a date.

Neither of us
Drink coffee.
A beginning
Of discovering
Many common
Preferences and
Now it seems
Like fate.

You share your
Profile direct.
I excitedly burst

With joy.
A reader of
Mary Oliver
Poems.
Now I know
You're the One
WildGeesemo11,
Magical attraction,
What bliss.

All the way
Down we love.
Inside out,
Upside Down,
Right side up.
Accepting,
Embracing
That first sweet kiss.

How warm your
Hand felt,
A glove
Made for
Mine.

Beautiful,
Handsome
Deep voice
Morning, evening,

Candles glowing
In a line.

Generously giving
Your time,
Attention,
Listening ear,
Insightful awareness
Straight from
Your full heart.

Brilliant mind,
Committed to things
Working,
Finding new pathways,
Solutions to
Puzzles that
Perplex.
Passionate for
Serving others
It's your art.

Those who
Serve you know
Because your gratitude
Gets expressed.
Seeking out waiters,
Waitresses,
Employees,

With thanks,
Praise.

Excellent
Adventures.
Laughing
Bonding
Dancing
Hiking
Moving.
Siting at
The lake in
Sun
Rays.

Joining our
Lives on
Magical
Mountain
North
Carolina,
We live
Golden
Bonus Round.

Unconditionally
Loving, Accepting
Generous
Affectionate

Self-aware
Tender
Caring
Acts of
Kindness
All around.

Five days
Five weeks
Five years
A lifetime.
I choose you
To hold and
Stand beside me.
My Love.
Here, now
Witnessing
Free to Be
All our days.

A perfect
Match with
Complimenting
Ways.
Soulful Love
Our Universe
Namaste
Namaste
Namaste.

Inside My Heart

With rapt
Attention
I see you
Fully.

I feel your
Calming energy
Deep in
The
Core of
Me.

I breathe
You inside
My heart.

I taste
Your kisses
On my forehead
Mouth

Fingers
Thighs
Toes

Delicious.

Our Love

You, beautiful spiritual teacher.
From you
I am learning to receive healthy love,
Heart, body, soul, being.
Breathe in your kindness,
Compassion, peace.
Breathe out laughter,
Babbling love stories.
Dancing in innocence, a flower
Gently blooming.
Seeing you, seeing me through Love's eyes
As the Universe intended.
Look up in wonder,
Awe at a sky.
Wispy, puffy, orange, purple streaked clouds.
Pure perfect expansion.
Awakened life force.
Give, be, welcome.
Born fresh from old wisdom.
Cherish
Our love.

Radiant

I feel your love
Because it lives
Inside of me
All intertwined
With mine.

The sky, the moon,
The flowing network
Of pathways leading
To my heart.
The interstellar
Vastness of stars,
Galaxies and
Worlds beyond
Beyond.

Rippling with
Ecstasy.
An entire energy
Field
Free and wild,

Sensuous and erotic,
Deep and wide,
Warm and soft,
Firm and strong,
Gentle and lilting,
Twinkling and shining.

Pulsing and bursting,
Breathing breathless,
Rolling belly laughing,
Dancing naked in the sunshine.
Running by deer,
Short grasses, ignored grasses,
Colorful, vibrant flowers,
Full trees,
And waterfalls.
Hearts being
Souls.
Minds being
Free.

Sweet Love

Sitting on a bench in
A park bursting with
Roses.
Looking at the
White fluff, puff
Formations
inside
a luminous bowl of blue.
Blooms glorious
In their
Shades of pink
Red, fuchsia.

Breathing in the
Gentle, unassuming
Presence of you.
A butterfly
Alighting on a
Petal, soft and
velvety

Like the ear
Of my dog.

Silent musings at the back
Brain where eight tracks
Of thought flow.

Side strokes of
Insight.
Dynamic, passionate
Pulsing, fluttering.
Dad jokes of
Laughter.

Do you know how to listen
from the caverns of
A hollowed out
Overflowing
Soul?

Do you know the
Watery words that fill
The barren quarry?

You live
Like a miracle
Of unwavering
Unrelenting

Streams of refreshing
Rain, beams of
Sunshine that
Quench and
Kiss a new day.

Wonderful Flavors

Have you sampled all the flavors of
Ice cream?
All the sweet ways
Compassion reveals itself?
A genuine smile from a cherished one
Lights up his entire face.
Twinkling, sparkling,
Sunlight reflections,
On a lake.
No need to squint or don sunglasses.
This is a glorious sight
For hungry, lonely, aching eyes.

A soft touch on the small of your back
Gently guiding you to a parked car.
A door being opened so you can
Step into many adventures together.
An offering of yogurt, nuts, a snack
From a kind man, your date for the evening.

Sitting on a bench mesmerized
By scents, the delight of
Gorgeous roses in a garden.
The arms of beloved ones
Wrapped around each other.
Torsos meet
In peace, warmth, comfort
Rhythmically
Meeting
Inhales of gratitude,
Exhales of grace,
Anticipating hearts beating.

You cannot imagine
Anywhere else you'd
Rather be except
Maybe an ice cream shop,
Where
Blood, Sweat, and Tears
Well known in your body,
Plays
"You've Made Me So Very Happy"
And then "Sexual Healing"
Like a current soundtrack swells
as
Bubbling laughter skips, gallops,
Joyfully dances in the air of freshly made
Waffle cones.

Astonished you suddenly
Realize you've
Walked a rocky road
As you scoop up
Heaping spoonfuls to your
Parting, once pursed lips,
Long ago parched mouth.
Experiencing the sweet,
The savory, the cold,
The crunch, the saltiness
Of knowing the
True taste of
Love in many of its
Wonderful flavors.

EXPANSIVE

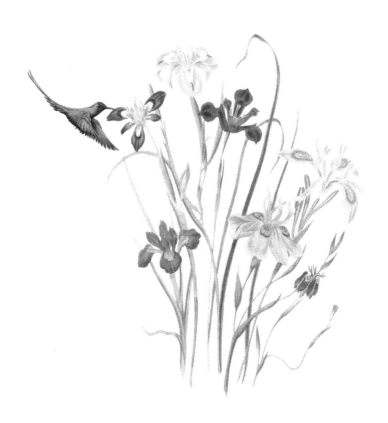

A Hundred Ways to Let Go

May the silent epidemic of shame be healed in the light of transparency, radical honesty, remorse, and fresh, healthy interactions.

May the amygdala of primitive survival strategies shrink as the human desire to thrive creates new pathways and possibilities for creative expression, caring, collaboration, and contribution.

May suppression of emotions end as we discover safe ways to express grief, anger, and loss without hurting ourselves or other people.

May oppression in all its forms implode as the groundswell for freedom, justice, and dignity rise strong.

May we shred limiting beliefs about ourselves and other human beings.

An Awakened Vision for the World

A world where emotional and relational maturity is celebrated by many people.

A world where people have a rich, deep, and wide experience of emotional wellness and can model emotional health for children of all ages-from infancy through the teenage years.

A world where people listen from the heart; quiet presence becomes celebrated reverently by as many people as possible.

A world where curiosity, creativity, collaboration, and contribution rise strong and transcend competition and comparisons.

A world where human beings experience their innate dignity, worth, and valuable presence here; human beings know their right to exist, to hear, see and value other people and to be heard, seen, and valued for their unique gifts, perspectives.

A world where honesty, kindness, radical empathy, and compassion are valued human character qualities that can be and are cultivated in the human spirit.

A world where being human means being multi-gifted, multifaceted; where an entire cornucopia, a colorful tapestry of life transcends a bifurcated mindset.

A world of rich biodiversity in the natural world and the human world in balance and harmony-living in balance and harmony in a reverent interconnected web of life.

A world abundant with love, possibility, beautiful sentient beings of all types.

Cold Rain

Running
Breathing
Layers
Legs tingling.

Core covered,
Face red,
Gloved hands
Warm.

Wind blows,
Intensifies.
Sweat cold
Clinging.

Seeping through
Layers of skin,
Resting on
The bark of
Bones.

Mist on
Mountains,
Shining With
Water.
Leaves flattened
In a splattering of
Red, deep red,
Eggplant, yellow, gold, and rusty orange.

The leaves all belong.
None takes another
For granted or wishes another harm.
They form a blanket,
A rich, diverse tapestry
Nestling the earth, soil,
Puddles and birdbaths.

Let's be like leaves,
Forming a human quilt
Of loving kindness,
Dignity, respect
A warm embrace
For all that is
Sacred and
Moving in the
Cold rain.

Hold Space

Someone
Somewhere
Loves
The Person
You Loathe.
Someone
Somewhere
Loathes
The Person
You Love.

Are we not
All messy
Mixtures of
Warmth, Saltiness,
Rosy, glowing,
Unsightly
Missteps,
Miscues,
Mistakes?

What does it
Mean to
Meet people
In their dark
Spaces of
Hurt,
Howling?
To hold
Space for
That Possible
Appearance
Of a
Beautiful Love
Being
With fleeting
Bandwidth to
Sustain Sanity?

Can you patiently
Await the glimmer
Of treasured
Goodness wrapped
In layers of
Irrational thoughts
Caustic speech
Raging unawareness?
Where does your
Goodness reside?

Your love?
Compassion?

Cultivating
Gifts as
People
Whisperers.
Alchemists
Transmuting
Energies of Loathing
Into Love sweet love.
Can we become
Alchemists
For One
Another?
May we,
Please?

Swept Under the Rug

Sweeping under the rug
Emotional dishonesty,
Ugly dark truths,
Resentments,
Insecurities,
Creates a lumpy,
Bumpy,
Disorienting walk across
What may never have been
A soft, cushioned, plush,
Shag carpet of
Privilege.

Lies and fear,
Historic invented
Constructs that demean
Many and elevate the few
Ultimately destroy the
Foundation of a
Common core

Of shared humanity
Through birth, maturation,
Death.

Collateral damage to
Human souls' need for
Empathy, love, dignity.
The hate you give away is
The hate you've allowed to
Fester,
Pus, and ooze inside
Old, unhealed wounds,
From a fake, distorted
Illusion of entitlement
That you got handed on
A Poo Poo Platter with a
Side of unquestioned
Ignorance.
You eat from the hand
That beat the shit out of you.
You trust in something outside
Yourself that isn't even real.
When did your faith cease to
Call you to love?
To love your enemies as yourself?
To turn the other cheek?
To cast the first stone
Only if you have not ever
Sinned?

Speaking Dreams

Radiant bold presence
Sparks
Words spoken,
Written from the heart of
Experience.

Wisdom ripened in
Rich fertile soils,
Raw, organic nutrients of
Imperfect,
Beautiful lives.

Nourishment to
Touch invisible threads
Of soft, tender, tough
Feelings.

Fresh
Awakenings in
Mind
Body.

Hope tingles
in the
Soul of
Humanity.

Teach Us

Mother Nature, teach us
To set down
Weapons of competition,
Jealousy, hate, greed,
Resentments against one another.
No tree is so foolish as to set its branches
Against one another
As swords of death.
Yet, humans do this in
A flash of incomprehensible fury.

The idea of a flower waits
Underneath,
Patient before pushing
Topsoil,
Green shoots of springtime.
A tight bud awaits
Perfect whispered wind kisses,
Tear drops of rain,
A slow unfurling,

Full blooming,
Colorful
Magnificence.

Crocuses, daffodils, roses, irises,
Day lilies, orchids
Do not sweat,
Toil around the clock,
Anxious about their worth,
Dignity,
Right to belong.

Sentient beings listen to natural rhythms
Eat the perfect amount of nutrition,
Drink water to
Quench their thirst.

Dolphins leap
Joyfully breaching,
No standing on a
Tipping scale
Crimson with shame.

Mother Nature teach us
Cycles, harmony, balance,
Ways to bring our bodies,
Hearts, souls into alignment
As vibrant, healthy expressions
Of Life.

Break Through

Bursting through the surface.
An imaginary seal between surf, cold air,
After swimming too long among
predatory sharks lustfully hunting
Shiny illusions that distract from
Deeper hungers.
Teeth grinding
Resentments
Birthed inside
Womb Abandonment,
Instigate Fear
Feeding frenzies,
Hide insecurities, lies
their own and yours.

Escape the dark
Depths of the ocean.
Flutter finned feet
Through kelp,
Schools of fish,

Towards the sun warmed
Sparkling bubbles,
Seafoam.
Body aching for
That very next
Inhale.
Feet
Shifting,
Sinking wet,
Warm sands of
Slipping time.

You were not meant
To remain forever in the depths
Of a dark bottomless place.

You were meant to
Break
Through
Expand gorgeous
Wings and
Soar far
Above the sea.

Possibilities

See beyond the packaging
Of a person into the heart
Of hurts and hopes with
Compassion,
Quiet empathy,
Gentleness,
Glasses if you are
Nearsighted, farsighted.
Can you witness the beauty, grief,
Loss, fatigue, spark, sass,
Radiance?

Look closely,
Patiently like
You are watching
Baby turtles emerge from their
Shells; a
Mother black bear foraging,
Coaxing her cubs up a tree;
A tiny hummingbird resting briefly
On a dead tree branch then

Whirring its wings in hovering
Flight at the edge of a
Flower filled with deliciousness,
Delight.

What awakens inside
When you observe, feel,
Sense from a soft in the
Sockets view?

Who could others become
When they are in your
Loving
Presence?

Human Wondering

Does hot coffee
With cream
Taste different
In your mouth?

What about cold
Water or bursting
Blueberries, sweet,
Tangy?

Doesn't a lover's kiss feel
Warm, tender,
Wet, sensuous, liberating
on your lips?

Do socks not make your
Feet feel safe, cozy
On a cold, autumn night?

Can you not feel the sun
On your face no matter

Your complexion, lines,
Wrinkles, shade, tone,
Creases?
Do you not look into a starlit
Night sky and notice the sliver
Glow of the moon?

Does your body not
Heave and grieve like mine?
Doesn't your belly
Digest food?
Your lungs expand with
Each breath?
When you hold a beloved one's hand
does this not soothe your wild,
fluttering heart?
Do we not all know death,
Birth, sweat, and salty tears?
My Pain, Your Joy
Your Hurts, My Love.
Our
Humanity.

Common Senses

Back muscles ache.
Hunger pangs.
A stuffed, bloated
Tummy, eating
Feelings of hurt, loss, grief.

Mind busy blathering
Thoughts distract
From wobbly knees,
Heat of a cracked heart.
Cool breath inhale,
Hot puff anger exhale.

Fingers touching
Soft skin, a beloved pet's fur,
A fuzzy blanket.
Contracted toes,
Relaxed face.
Full bladder
Urge To pee. Thirsty.

Feet bare in the sand,
Dirt, hot pavement.

Walking on top of trash,
Pieces of glass,
A plastic child's toy,
Warm, squishy mud
A lake bottom,
Wet ankles.
A wisp of hair dances
Near the corner of a
Teary eye.

A cool wind blows
Creating goosebumps
On arms.
Staring with awe,
A breathtaking sunset.

Salivating with
Thoughts of eating
Savory, sweet, creamy,
Crunchy, piping hot
Indian, Mexican,
Thai, Indonesian
French,
Dutch
Root Beer Float
Cuisine.

An accidental cut.
Skin stings,
Bleeds blood red.
Invisible oxygen
Penetrates
Previously
Blue
Veined life
Energy.

Scent of fear.
Tingles of excitement.
Flush of embarrassment.
Tickle of laughter.
Pounding heart.

Do we not
Share
Common
Senses?

Wishes

To hug
Children,
Grandchildren
In strong, soft
Arms in the
Many minutes
A chocolate cake
Takes to
Bake.

To hold hands
With dear
Friends
Feeling the warmth
Of skin touch
As they
Grieve.

To trust
That
Deaths

Protests
Dangerous Decisions
Violence
Systemic Oppression
Implode
Giving
Rise
To
Transformation
Transcendence
Equality
Wellness
Justice
Peace
Oneness.

To make
Mundane choices
Standing, gazing at
Favorite nutritious foods, clear
Preferences in a
Grocery aisle. A simple
Joy never again to
Be taken for
Granted.

For large and
Small gatherings of
People.

Being
Able to look, to
Breathe in
Beautiful faces, smiles,
Shining eyes,
Tearful.

How exceptional
What used to seem
So ordinary.

For a Celebration of Humanity
Multifaceted
Multitalented
Complex
Diverse
Rich, Glorious
Expressions of Uniqueness,
Connected in
The Heart of
Grief, Tenderness,
Love, Compassion,
Courage, Dignity,
Empathy, and humility.
Awakened in Conscious
Responsive
Contribution.

For Soul Freedom
Soaring,
Unbounded, unleashed,
Untamed,
Unwavering, unrelenting
Everywhere.

For a planet
That revers life
Itself, humming
In harmony with grasses,
Trees, bees, bears, deer, snakes,
Turtles, birds, glorious
Blue hydrangea bushes,
Purple iris, lakes, rivers,
Mountains, oceans.

For a restorative night's
Sleep knowing in
Your weary bones
That radical imagination
Remains
Essential
For
Our
Extraordinary
Existence.

The Search

Last night
I dreamt
I was looking for
My higher self.

Or was I
Searching for
A Backpack?

My higher self
Might
Be in the
Backpack!

Let me unzip
And feel around.
Are you fuzzy
And flexible?
Slippery and
Soft?

Do you feel
Like pencils,
Markers, books,
Glue
Stuck to
Stardust?

Can I read
You like
An open
Book of
Hilarious
Poems,
The black squiggles
Pointing
To the wisdom
Of the ages?

Ah, the weight
Of you fell
To the bottom.
Crumpled
Love notes,
Fuzz balls.

Crushed, tiny,
Wrapped gifts
Of kindness
Compassion

Courage
Creativity
Can now
Be Opened.

Welcome
To the Bonus
Round of
Being alive
Unfettered
Free.

Cherish Awakened Awareness

An experiencer inside
The Mindbody
All your life.
Gazing out through eyeballs,
Sensing
Eight, nine, ten gatherers
Of how human software
Hardware
Ticks, tocks.
Bearing witness
To thoughts,
Feelings,
Rumblings,
Imaginative wonderings,
Wanderings.
Teller of stories
That got recorded.
Movie scenes on a
Projector Screen.
Laugh, cry,
Cringe,

Shake, fume, whistle,
Swoon, cheer.
Roll down hills of soft grass
Conscious Holder
Of human being.
Taste a crisp, tart, sweet apple
Crunching
Juiciness inside a warm
Familiar
Untamed wilderness.
Recognize another
Face disappeared.
Lids gently blink.
Shutter closes
windows of
Hearts.

A beautiful, beaming
Radiant lover of every single
Invisible inhale of breath,
Soft breeze
Greeting the skin.
Delicious kisses
Melting moments
One flowing
Into the Next One.

Cherish

Awakened awareness
That sees you beyond
Vagaries, vulgarities
Vacant lost lots and inside
Rainbows of thawed
Dreams coming
Alive
All of them.
All of them.
A parade of joy
Diamonds excavated
By the only hand
That could touch
That sacred place of
Beauty
Inside
Your
Abundant
Heart.

A Grateful Heart

To the many different people from all parts of my life with whom I've been blessed to cross paths. Thank you for the rich lessons you brought to me about being human, healing, loving, and living free.

To you, dear reader, thank you.

About the Author

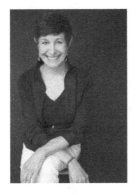

The founder of Cherish Your World, Laura Staley passionately supports people thriving by guiding them to a holistic transformation of space, heart, and life. Laura knows that there's a relationship between the conditions of our homes or workplaces and the quality of our lives. Trained and certified with the Western School of Feng Shui and seasoned by two decades of working with a variety of clients, Laura uses her intuition and expertise to empower her clients to produce remarkable results in their lives. Her trifecta of serving people includes speaking, writing, and compassionate listening. She serves clients in central Ohio, western North Carolina, and on Zoom.

As a columnist with BizCatalyst360, an award-winning, multi-media digest, Laura writes personal essays focused on self-discovery, feng shui, emotional health, and transformations from the inside out. Laura is the published author of three books: *Live Inspired, Let Go Courageously and Live with Love: Transform Your Life with Feng Shui,* and the *Cherish Your World Gift Book of 100 Tips to Enhance Your Home and Life.* Her essay "He Had Me at Mary Oliver" published in the best-selling anthology, *Crappy to Happy: Sacred Stories of Transformational Joy* by Rev. Ariel Patricia & Kathleen O'Keefe-Kanavos.

Prior to creating her company, Laura worked as a fulltime parent and an assistant professor at Ohio Wesleyan University. She earned a Ph.D. in political science from The Ohio State University. Her joys in life include laughing with loved ones, dancing, reading, meditating, running, being in nature, and listening to music she loves. She resides in Black Mountain, NC.